WHAT NURSES KNOW…

D I A B E T E S

WHAT NURSES KNOW...

DIABETES

Rita Girouard Mertig
MS, RNC, CNS, DE

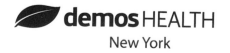

demos HEALTH
New York

ISBN: 978-1-932603-98-9
Visit our web site at www.demoshealth.com

Acquisitions Editor: Noreen Henson
Cover Design: Steve Pisano
Compositor: NewGen
Printer: Hamilton Printing

Medical information provided by Demos Health, in the absence of a visit with a healthcare professional, must be considered as an educational service only. This book is not designed to replace a physician's independent judgment about the appropriateness or risks of a procedure or therapy for a given patient. Our purpose is to provide you with information that will help you make your own healthcare decisions.

The information and opinions provided here are believed to be accurate and sound, based on the best judgment available to the authors, editors, and publisher, but readers who fail to consult appropriate health authorities assume the risk of any injuries. The publisher is not responsible for errors or omissions. The editors and publisher welcome any reader to report to the publisher any discrepancies or inaccuracies noticed.

Library of Congress Cataloging-in-Publication Data
A catalog record for this book is available from the Library of Congress.

Special discounts on bulk quantities of Demos Health books are available to corporations, professional associations, pharmaceutical companies, health care organizations, and other qualifying groups. For details, please contact:

Special Sales Department
Demos Medical Publishing
11 W. 42nd Street
New York, NY 10036
Phone: 800-532-8663 or 212-683-0072
Fax: 212-941-7842
E-mail: rsantana@demosmedpub.com

Made in the United States of America
10 11 12 13   5 4 3 2 1

About the Author

Rita Girouard Mertig, MS, RNC, CNS, DE has been a registered nurse for 43 years with a Master of Science degree. She has taught nursing in a variety of programs and recently retired after 21 years from teaching in an associate degree nursing program in which she also taught nutrition. Rita also has had type 1 diabetes for 25 years and has used an insulin pump for 15 years. She currently volunteers at CrossOver Ministries clinic where she teach classes and conducts one-on-one sessions on weight management and diabetes management for clients with minimal ability to pay for services. During the 1980s and 90s, Rita led a support group for people with diabetes who were using insulin under the auspices of the American Diabetes Association, Richmond, VA chapter, and has also served on the board of directors. She has previously authored two books, *Teaching Nursing in an Associate Degree Program* and *The Nurses' Guide to Teaching Diabetes Self-Management* both published by Springer Publishing Company.

WHAT NURSES KNOW...

Nurses hold a critical role in modern health care that goes beyond their day-to-day duties. They share more information with patients than any other provider group, and are alongside patients twenty-four hours a day, seven days a week, offering understanding of complex health issues, holistic approaches to ailments, and advice for the patient that extends to the family. Nurses themselves are a powerful tool in the healing process.

What Nurses Know gives down-to-earth information, addresses consumers as equal partners in their care, and explains clearly what readers need to know and wants to know to understand their condition and move forward with their lives.

Contents

Foreword

I met Rita many years ago while volunteering with the American Diabetes Association (ADA), Richmond, Virginia Chapter. At the time I was a Diabetes Educator at a local hospital. Because I have had type 1 diabetes since 1969, I went to nursing school in order to become a Diabetes Educator. I wanted to work with "people like myself". I was delighted and flattered when Rita asked me to write the foreword to this book. Rita has always seen what the person with diabetes has needed: guidance and support, be it technical or emotional. This book provides much of the information one needs to get started on the right foot to managing their diabetes.

While volunteering with the ADA I started treating my diabetes using the MiniMed 504S insulin pump. I had started many of my patients on pumps and thought it was time I did the same. This began my journey to specializing in pump therapy. About a year after starting on the pump I organized an insulin pump support group. All "pumpers" needed the emotional support and camaraderie. Also, they needed to know how others handled life events such as Thanksgiving and wedding receptions. The conversations that took place were invaluable. Eventually I went to work for MiniMed, now Medtronic Diabetes.

Earlier this year I returned for a college reunion. I learned many of my college friends had developed type 2 diabetes and were struggling to gain control over their disease. Many of them had not been sent for any education, which I believe is a disservice and a guarantee for failure. Also, most were not instructed or told to monitor their glucose, another disservice. Without knowing your glucose level how do you know if what you are doing is working? Diabetes is a patient managed disease. A physician can only tell you what needs to be done. It is then your responsibility to do it. But without the knowledge of "how" to do it, one cannot achieve success.

If every person with newly diagnosed diabetes were provided Rita's book they would have the stepping stones to succeeding in the management of their diabetes.

—Carolyn Allen, BA, BSN, RN, CDE

Acknowledgments

I would like to thank the following people who made it possible for me to write this book.

Noreen Henson, Director of DemosHealth, who was so generous with her time, advice, and encouragement; thanks for reading each chapter to make sure I was on track with other books in this series. My family, who gave of their time generously and were always willing to rearrange planned family events to suit my writing schedule; I owe them my sanity. My adult daughters, Karen and Kelley, who generously gave me the benefit of their wisdom. Kelley, a budding author herself, has spent many hours and days putting up with my handwriting, changes with odd directions, and typing chapters; thanks for saving me a lot of time and advising me on my computer concerns. My husband, Bob, who took over most of the cooking and grocery shopping, despite his full-time job, so I could pursue my goal of completing the manuscript. To the many clients at CrossOver Ministries Clinic who listened to and followed my instructions on nutrition and diabetes self-management; you helped me to understand where you were coming from and what you needed from a diabetes educator. You may recognize yourselves in some of my vignettes.

−Rita Girouard Mertig

Introduction

Is there life after diagnosis? When I was diagnosed with diabetes in my late 30s, I had my doubts. I went through all of Dr. Elizabeth Kübler-Ross's "stages of grief" (denial, anger, bargaining, despair, and finally acceptance) which are as pertinent to loss of perceived health as they are to loss of a body part or of life itself when a terminal diagnosis is given. In my mind, the plans I had made for my life, my family, my career, would never be realized. Not me! I wasted three months of my life in denial, eating very few carbohydrates, exercising after every meal, and seeing another physician for an alternative diagnosis, all to no avail. I was also angry with everyone I knew who smoked, was overweight, or who did not exercise. I was also very angry with God. Why me? I took care of my body and look at the thanks I got.

When I finally decided that "Yes, it is me but—," the bargaining began. OK, as long as I don't have to take insulin, I can manage life with diabetes. Meanwhile, I was reading everything I could get my hands on and asking my physician a million questions.

This was back in the days before widespread use of glucose monitors. Human insulin had just come on the market, and there were only three oral medications for diabetes, drugs that are rarely used today. I was prescribed the maximum dose of the strongest one. When this drug failed to decrease my blood sugar, I was put on insulin. I gave myself my first shot of insulin in the examination room under the supervision of a nurse. I did it perfectly, having given many injections to others during my nursing career. I had also taught and supervised many student nurses giving injections for several years. However, after this first injection, I cried for twenty to thirty minutes. It didn't hurt, but my denial was over. I could no longer pretend my diabetes pills were vitamins. My bargaining had failed. I did have diabetes and would be giving myself insulin injections for the rest of my probably shortened life. It might also mean I'd be on dialysis, perhaps blind and missing a few toes or worse before I finally died. To put it mildly, I was very depressed.

I don't know what helped me to turn my attitude around, to finally accept my fate and work at making the best of what I considered to be a dismal future. Maybe it was the hope I received from all of my research about diabetes management. Maybe it was my husband's faith in my ability to overcome adversity. However, I think what really helped me come to grips with this diagnosis was that I had to be a positive role model for my children just in case I had passed on this hereditary disease. I had to demonstrate that there was "life after diagnosis."

We all experience the stages of grief differently. For example, depression may be experienced as a low blow, as it was in my situation, and acceptance may lead you to decide how you want to live the rest of your life. By getting this book and reading it, you have moved in the right direction toward developing an action plan for you. When you experience anger you may want to use that anger to get energized. I like to say, "I can't waste a good mad." Anger often got me to start writing a new book. It did not need to relate to diabetes or anything that I was experiencing. It simply got me energized to do something besides feel sorry for myself. I wrote things like "slogans to live by". I started a book on raising children. I worked on remaking some of my favorite recipes to reduce the fat, sugar, and calories so someone with diabetes could eat them. I also began several books about my journey with diabetes and it didn't matter that I never finished them. What mattered was that I used the energy anger produces and it provided me with a new focus. You might want to take up a new hobby or sport or something else that makes you feel more in control of your life. Think about it.

I don't mean to imply that the past 25 years have been a walk in the park because they haven't been. Living with diabetes is complex and requires renewed dedication at frequent intervals. In this book I ask many questions and, hopefully, provide answers that are relevant to your life or the life of a friend or family member. These are the questions I have asked healthcare professionals and myself over the years. I have also included questions I have heard from others as I pursued my nursing career, taught student nurses the basics of diabetes, and counseled others who may be as confused, discouraged, frightened or depressed as I was after being diagnosed with diabetes. I start each chapter with one or more of these questions and try to answer them with as much detail as I can. I have included a resource list of Web sites in the back of the book if you need more or different information.

Chapter 1 deals with the basics of diabetes, what it is and how it affects people who have it. It is important to understand the types of diabetes, how they differ, how to prevent them especially with regard to type 2 diabetes, and how each is treated. It should answer questions about how this happened to you and what you might look forward to in the rest of the book as to what information you need. I also discuss the genetics of each type of diabetes in this chapter. The information here may give you questions to ask your doctor or healthcare professional. My advice is that you have a pad of paper handy. As you think of questions during the reading of this book or at any time in the future you should write them down and take them with you when you see a healthcare practitioner. As you walk in to see this professional with your pad in hand, it will alert this person to the fact that you have questions. He/she should not attempt to hurry you knowing you have questions to ask and should allow time to answer them. Otherwise you might get flustered, forget the questions, or not ask them in the way that you meant to ask. It is also wise to bring along a friend or family member especially in the beginning. This should be someone supportive who will also hear the same instructions you do and can help you with recall in the future. This should be a person you trust who will not nag you about some of the things that you may or may not want to have thrown back at you. Often this may be a friend and not a family member. No matter who it is, bringing somebody with you is always a good idea.

Chapter 2 covers nutrition and answers the question "What can I eat?" That was my basic question after I was diagnosis. What am I going to cook for supper? It may seem minor, but it was quite dramatic. I had no idea what I should or should not eat despite the fact that I was a nurse. I decided to simply prepare what I had planned figuring that it was probably an OK meal. I obviously knew that I should not serve dessert until I figured this out. I saw a registered dietician for more specific information and bought a couple of cookbooks to get a feel for the diabetic diet. I ended up realizing that it was pretty much the same diet I normally served my family and that what I had eaten in the past was NOT the reason I have diabetes now. This may or may not be true for you. What I advise is to avoid preparing a separate meal for you. This practice is very discouraging, makes you angry, and feeling very different and alone. What everybody else is eating should be healthy food. I came to the conclusion that I needed a healthy diet. Why would I serve my family anything different?

Chapter 3 discusses physical activity which does not have to be what most people would consider exercise. You don't have to jog, swim, or lift weights. Physical activity is physical activity. This chapter will help you identify various types of movement and the parameters with which to view any physical activity, whether it is cleaning the house, walking the dog, or planting a garden. These parameters are very important if you are taking insulin or any kind of medication that that increases the amount of insulin your body produces.

Medications are discussed in Chapter 4. Whether you are on pills or shots, your questions about how these drugs work, when they should be taken, and any side effects you should be aware of are answered. I've also included how to do an internet search of new drugs as they come on the market.

Chapter 5 is my favorite chapter since it deals with glucose monitoring. Keeping track of blood sugar levels can be very frustrating. The questions here include: Why is my blood sugar so high or low? What do I do with the numbers on my meter? I also discuss what raises and lowers blood glucose levels.

The focus of Chapter 6 is about chronic complications. They may or may not occur depending upon how well you make the necessary changes to your lifestyle. Chronic complications like hypertension and heart disease, which are very common in anybody with diabetes, are covered. I also discuss eye disease, kidney disease, diseases of the nervous system, and gum disease. Prevention is the name of the game but I also talk about how these complications are currently being treated.

Pregnancy with diabetes or with gestational diabetes is the focus of Chapter 7. The blood sugar goals are lower than in the non-pregnant state and for good reason. The health of the mother and the fetus are involved. If type 1 or type 2 diabetes precedes pregnancy, then good glucose control prior to getting pregnant is very important. How to do this is also covered in this chapter.

Chapter 8 discusses emotions and covers the different effects depression, anger, frustration, and stress have on blood sugar. These emotions accompany the diagnosis of diabetes, and/or may happen down the road even if you work at making the changes this diagnosis demands. When emotions complicate the normalization of blood sugar levels, you need to know how to gain back control.

Chapter 9 provides information on getting the help you need. This is very important to your success in living well with diabetes. Many healthcare professionals are well versed in diabetes care but their approach to diabetes and yours may be different. Your healthcare practitioner needs to work with you and give you the knowledge and understanding concerning how you want to live your life. If you do not feel that your needs are being met, it is really important to find another practitioner in the same practice or in another practice. You need help in dealing with the many aspects of diabetes care unique to you. You need to trust your healthcare provider, so it is imperative to be assertive and to find what you need in a healthcare professional. Again bring a friend or family member. It will encourage you to ask questions, make decisions, and get the care that you want.

I have also included a chapter specifically for friends and family members since their concerns may or may not be the same as yours. I have added a list of what to say and what not to say and a Web site that explains this in more detail. I think that a person with a chronic illness, particularly something like diabetes, will bring out the best and the worst in people who are trying to be helpful. This may move you to share this chapter with the friends and family that you need for support but who are inadvertently not doing or saying the things that you need them to do or say.

Since diabetes is a life-long illness, I discuss how to stay motivated in the last chapter. Preventing burnout and what to do if it occurs is very important in your success at living with this disease.

The Resources section in the back of the book covers mostly Web resources. However, phone numbers and addresses have been provided where applicable, enabling you, your friends, and family to obtain information or more specific information in each area. I have provided online sources such as Baja Bob in California where you can order sugar-free drink mixers if you want to have a cocktail. There are also other resources for flavorings for coffee or to put on ice cream, etc.

The Glossary should be particularly useful for explaining medical terms used in this book. Please use it to increase your understanding.

The diagnosis of diabetes may be for you, as it was for me, a wake-up call. Just like going to college, getting married, having children, and a host of other of life's changes, your life, now that you have diabetes, will never be the same—and that might be a good thing.

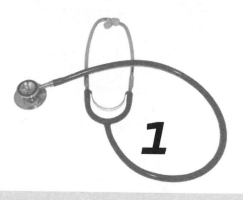

Diabetes—What Is It?

I was diagnosed with gestation[al] diabetes during the pregnancy with my youngest child. Five years later I lost 15 pounds without even trying, was going to the bathroom every few hours day and night, always thirsty and hungry for sweets. What bothered me the most was my new blurred vision. My doctor did test and told me I had diabetes. He prescribed the max dose of Diabenese and that didn't hardly touch the glucose level. I am very confused. He is treating me like a type 2 diabetic because I am 39? I have no family members with diabetes and I'm not overweight. Am I a type 2 or a type 1? RITA

If you or a friend or family member has been diagnosed with diabetes, you probably have many questions and concerns like Rita's. First it is important to define diabetes and explore the ins and outs of how and why this happened. I hope this chapter will answer some of your questions. In the next few chapters I will discuss what you can do to control blood sugar levels with healthy eating; exercise; and medication, if needed. Glucose monitoring, discussed in Chapter 5, is the most useful way to follow how successful your efforts are.

The Centers for Disease Control and Prevention defines diabetes mellitus as a group of chronic diseases marked by high levels of blood glucose resulting from defects in insulin production, insulin action, or both. The bad news is that uncontrolled high blood sugar can lead to complications of the eyes, kidneys, heart, blood vessels, and nerves. The good news is that we can do something to prevent these. In this chapter I will describe the various types of diabetes and discuss how they are different from each other and how we can prevent or control this potentially devastating disease.

It is helpful to remember that you are not alone. In the fall of 2007 the Centers for Disease Control and Prevention estimated that nearly twenty-four million adults and children in the United States have diabetes mellitus. Of this number, 17.9 million are diagnosed, thus leaving 5.7 million, or 25% of the total, as yet undiagnosed. Before changes to the diagnostic criteria were made in 1997, it was once estimated that half of all persons with diabetes did not know they had the disease. The 1997 American Diabetes Association (ADA) diagnostic and classification criteria lowered the fasting blood sugar from 140 mg/dl (milligrams per deciliter) to 126 mg/dl, resulting in many more people being diagnosed and treated. The goal was to identify and treat as many persons as possible to prevent long-term complications. It seems that what you don't know can and will hurt you.

How Insulin Works

Insulin is a protein and a hormone secreted by the beta cells found throughout the pancreas. When blood sugar (*glucose*) rises after one consumes a meal, insulin is secreted to help glucose move into the cells of the body to be used as fuel. If there is more glucose than needed for cellular energy, insulin helps sugar fill storage places in the liver and the muscles of the arms and legs for later use. Glucose is stored here as *glycogen*. When the amount of glucose in the blood is greater than required by these two needs, the rest is stored in fat cells, causing weight gain. Another role of insulin is to prevent the liver from releasing stored glycogen when it is not needed. However, if there is a drop in blood sugars—for example, from prolonged exercise or a skipped meal—another pancreatic hormone, *glucagon*, is secreted to allow the stored glycogen to be released from the liver to maintain normal blood glucose levels. This is very important, because the cells of the brain and nervous system burn only glucose for energy. The rest of the body can function by burning fat and protein for energy in the absence of blood glucose, but the brain cannot.

HOW THE PANCREAS REGULATES BLOOD SUGAR

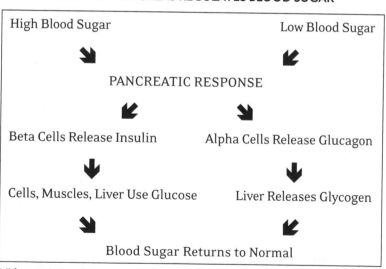

With permission from Mertig, RG, *The Nurse's Guide to Teaching Diabetes Self-Management*, Springer Publishing Company, LLC, New York, NY.

The beta cells that produce insulin and the alpha cells that produce glucagon are part of the *islets of Langerhans* that are scattered throughout the pancreas. This fact is important to remember as you read about the new islet cell transplantation being used to reverse type 1 diabetes. Another important fact is that, in a normal pancreas, only approximately one fourth of the beta cells are needed to keep blood sugars within normal range. The other three fourths may be called on when more insulin is needed, for example, when the blood glucose load from a meal is high; when stress and other hormones increase the release of stored glycogen; or when the body is fighting an infection or other physical condition, such as an injury or pregnancy. Only when the need for insulin outstrips the supply does blood sugar rise.

Classification of Diabetes

What is in a name? Well, as it turns out, quite a bit. The ADA has been reclassifying and renaming the types of diabetes over the years as more is understood about the pathology and causes of each. A major effort was made in 1997 to get rid of old and misleading terms. *Type 1 diabetes* is no longer called *juvenile diabetes* because people, such as myself, are being diagnosed in their 40s and older. Likewise, *type 2 diabetes* is not thought of as just *adult onset diabetes* because obese children as young as four years old meet the criteria. Also, treatment with insulin is not the deciding factor between type 1 and type 2 diabetes because insulin is but one of the many medications appropriately used to treat persons with type 2 diabetes.

The pathology that causes each type of diabetes is very different, which is why a person with type 2 diabetes cannot develop type 1 simply because he or she takes insulin to control blood sugar. The following table helps clarify the differences.

Type 1 diabetes is an autoimmune disease in that the body's own immune system attacks and destroys the beta cells of the

DIABETES CLASSIFICATIONS

	Cause	Fasting Blood Sugar	Heredity	Insulin Production
Normal		70–99 mg/dl		Normal
Prediabetes	Decreased insulin sensitivity	100–125 mg/dl	Very strong	Increased production
Type 1	Autoimmune destruction of beta cells	126 mg/dl & up	Not common	Very little
Type 2	Insulin resistance or inadequate amount of insulin	126 mg/dl & up	Very strong	Increased then decreased
Gestational diabetes	Placental hormones cause insulin resistance, insufficient insulin	Abnormal oral glucose tolerance test at 26–32 weeks	Very strong	Increased
Other (pancreatitis, pancreatic & other cancers, & some drugs)	Abnormal production of hormones causing insulin resistance	126 mg/dl & up	Sometimes	Decreased

With permission from Mertig, RG, *The Nurse's Guide to Teaching Diabetes Self-Management*, Springer Publishing Company, LLC, New York, NY.

pancreas. Thus, in a short span of time, from weeks to a few years, the body does not even have the minimum one fourth of beta cells functioning to prevent a rise in blood sugar.

Individuals with type 1 diabetes are not the persons who live for years with undiagnosed diabetes. They are diagnosed relatively

What Nurses Know ...

If you have type 1 diabetes, which is an autoimmune disease, there is a possibility that you may develop other autoimmune diseases, such as hypo- or hyperthyroidism; rheumatoid arthritis; systemic lupus erythematosis; Crohn's disease; and other, less well-known diseases. Your healthcare provider should periodically test you for thyroid conditions (the next most common autoimmune disease after type 1 diabetes).

quickly because they have the symptoms of a potentially life-threatening condition. When the body stops producing enough insulin, the cells are starved of their preferred fuel, glucose. The body then begins to burn fat, and then protein, for energy. The breakdown of fat produces fatty acids and ketones that begin to poison the body. The burning of fat and protein reduces the body's fat and lean muscle mass, causing a life-threatening weight loss. The body is literally wasting away because the cells have no way of getting to the ever-rising sugar in the blood without insulin to transport it past the cell wall. And if that were not bad enough, the high blood glucose increases the concentration, or thickness, of the blood, so water is pulled from cells and interstitial fluid (fluid around the cells) to dilute the sugar concentration in the blood. The kidneys then dump some of the excess sugar and water as "very sweet urine" (*glycosuria*). Without injections of insulin, the body and its cells become very dehydrated, to the point of multi-organ failure. Prior to the discovery of insulin in the early 1920s, children with this disease all died. Today, persons with type 1 diabetes account for five to ten percent of those with diabetes, and with lifestyle modifications, blood sugar control, and insulin injections they can live long, productive lives.

Type 2 diabetes, on the other hand, stems from cellular insulin resistance, not enough insulin produced to overcome this resistance, or a production of insulin that the body cannot use efficiently. Many cases comprise a combination of all three factors. Insulin resistance is often found in persons who are overweight or obese. Obese persons who have not inherited the gene for type 2 diabetes simply produce a large amount of insulin to overcome this resistance and maintain normal blood sugar levels. When type 2 diabetes runs in the family, obesity often results in a diagnosis. According to Christopher Saudek and Simeon Margolis, "About 80% of people with type 2 diabetes are overweight or obese, and the risk of type 2 diabetes rises as a person's weight increases." Because this form of diabetes has a strong genetic component, the population at risk for developing type 2 diabetes includes members of the following ethnic groups:

- African Americans
- Asian Americans
- Pacific Islanders, such as Hawaiians and Filipinos
- Native Americans (American Indians)
- Mexican Americans

In addition, all overweight and obese individuals have an increased risk of developing *metabolic syndrome*, the components of which include obesity, high cholesterol and triglycerides, high blood pressure, and insulin resistance. This syndrome affects at least one out of every five overweight people and increases their risk of being diagnosed with type 2 diabetes. If you are experiencing any of these components and are concerned that you might be developing type 2 diabetes, there is a test that can tell you your risk of developing type 2 in the next five years. The PreDx Diabetes Risk Score test, developed by Tethys Bioscience, measures seven biomarkers (chemical measurements of biological processes underlying type 2 diabetes) and calculates a prediagnosis risk score. It must be ordered by

What Nurses Know...

Type 2 diabetes is much more than just a "touch of sugar." It is as serious a disease as type 1 diabetes, and individuals with type 2 diabetes need to make the same concentrated effort to eat healthy foods and lose weight; increase activity level; and control blood sugar with medication, if needed.

your healthcare professional. To learn more about this test, go to http://predxdiabetes.com. Anyone with type 2 diabetes is at high risk for developing heart disease, hypertension, stroke, blood vessel problems leading to amputation, vision problems, kidney disease, and nervous system difficulties.

Another type of diabetes is *gestational diabetes mellitus* (GDM), which occurs only during pregnancy. It occurs in about three to ten percent of all pregnancies in the United States, resulting in at least 135,000 cases diagnosed each year. Ninety percent of all women who have pregnancies complicated by diabetes have GDM. Women who are overweight or obese, have a family history of type 2 diabetes, and/or are from one of the high-risk populations listed earlier have a much greater risk of developing GDM than the general population. Pregnancy and the resulting placental hormones cause some degree of insulin resistance in all women; however, a healthy pancreas is able to produce more and more insulin to keep blood sugars within normal range as the pregnancy advances. Today it is recommended that all but low-risk women be tested for GDM between 24 and 28 weeks of gestation, because controlling blood glucose during pregnancy enhances maternal and fetal health. Immediately after pregnancy, five to ten percent of women with GDM are found to have diabetes, usually type 2. The rest of these women have a forty to sixty percent risk of developing type 2 diabetes later in life, often within five to ten years of the pregnancy. You can read more about diabetes during pregnancy in Chapter 7.

There is a fourth classification of diabetes, termed "other," which includes individuals who have a diseased pancreas caused by cancer or infection and those with drug-induced high blood glucose, as is often the case in persons taking prescriptions for prednisone or other steroid medications. (A list of medications that increase blood sugar is provided in Chapter 5.)

In recent years we have heard a lot about *prediabetes*, a term used to alert both healthcare providers and clients to the fact that time is running out to prevent future cases of diabetes, heart disease, and stroke. Prior to developing type 2 diabetes, most clients have had difficulty with glucose control, perhaps for years. This includes a number of people who have metabolic syndrome. Research has shown that organ damage often begins during the prediabetes years. The normal fasting blood sugar level once was defined as 70-109 mg/dl, and an impaired fasting glucose level was identified as 110-125 mg/dl. In 2003, these criteria were lowered to help motive individuals with prediabetes to follow guidelines and prevent or delay the diagnosis of type 2 diabetes and long-term complications. These guidelines include weight loss, exercise, and lifestyle modifications. There are about fifty-seven million Americans diagnosed with prediabetes today. This is an increase from forty million in the 2005 statistics. As stated in the 2010 Johns Hopkins White Papers on Diabetes, "Without lifestyle changes or medication, many [individuals with prediabetes] will develop type 2 diabetes in the next 10 years." The hope is that, if forewarned, people with prediabetes will make the changes needed in diet and physical activity that will result in weight loss and lower fasting blood sugars to less than 100 mg/dl and that healthcare practitioners will be more concerned about the health consequences to their patients in the years prior to their official diagnosis of type 2 diabetes and help them prevent it from developing.

Diagnostic Criteria

Most people with diabetes are diagnosed with a fasting blood glucose of 126 mg/dl or higher or a nonfasting blood glucose of 200 mg/dl. In 2010, the ADA added an A1c of more than 6.5% to the diagnostic criteria. *Hemoglobin A1c*, or simply *A1c*, is a blood test that measures one's average blood sugar level over 2 to 3 months. To put this in perspective, a person without diabetes would have an A1c of 4 to 6%.

Current ADA recommendations for screening people without symptoms include a fasting blood sugar, an A1c, or a two-hour 75-g oral glucose tolerance test for all individuals forty-five years old and older and, if the results are normal, repeating one of these tests every three years. Screening should be done earlier than forty-five years and/or be done more frequently for individuals who have any of the following risk factors:

— Overweight body mass index (BMI; >25 kg/m^2)
— Habitually physically inactive
— First-degree relative with type 2 diabetes (parent, sibling, child)
— Member of a high-risk ethnic population (e.g., African American, Asian American, Pacific Islander, Native American, Mexican American)

What Nurses Know...

Common symptoms of diabetes that might indicate a blood glucose test is needed include excessive urination; excessive thirst; weight loss despite cravings for and eating sweets (type 1); fatigue; skin lesions that do not heal; repeat infection; and any end organ damage associated with chronic diabetic complication, particularly heart and nerve problems (type 2).

- Delivered a baby weighing >9 lbs or diagnosed with GDM
- Hypertensive (≥140/90 mm Hg)
- High-density lipoprotein ("good" cholesterol) <35 mg/dl and/ or triglyceride level >250 mg/dl
- Polycystic ovary syndrome
- On previous testing had impaired glucose tolerance or impaired fasting glucose
- Any other clinical condition associated with insulin resistance
- History of vascular disease

Because the incidence of type 2 diabetes in adolescents and children has increased dramatically in the last 10 years, children who meet the criteria listed next are thus at increased risk of developing type 2 diabetes in childhood and should be tested at puberty or age 10, whichever comes first, and retested every two years using a fasting blood sugar or an A1c blood test.

- Overweight (BMI >85th percentile for age and sex, weight for height >85th percentile, or weight >120% of ideal for height)

Plus any two of the following risk factors:

- Family history of type 2 diabetes in first- or second-degree relative
- Race/ethnicity (African American, Asian American, Pacific Islander, Native American, Mexican American)
- Signs of insulin resistance or conditions associated with insulin resistance (high blood pressure, high cholesterol, or polycystic ovary syndrome)

Children who have signs and symptoms of diabetes, such as excessive, pale urine; constant thirst; excessive cravings for sweets; and rapid, unintentional weight loss probably have type 1 diabetes and are in immediate danger of developing diabetic ketoacidosis, which can be life threatening.

GENETICS OF DIABETES

If you are concerned about the potential of passing on this disease, as I was, consider the following information from the ADA:

1. For both type 1 and type 2 diabetes you must inherit a predisposition to the disease.
2. As stated earlier, something in your environment must trigger the onset of diabetes. With type 1 it is probably a virus. Type 2 is generally precipitated by obesity and too little exercise, and it has a much greater genetic basis than type 1.
3. Women who develop GDM are more likely to have a family history of diabetes, especially on their mother's side, and be overweight prior to the pregnancy. Women who have had GDM have an increased risk of developing type 2 diabetes within ten years of the pregnancy.

Your child's risk for developing type 1 diabetes is as follows:

- The child of a man with type 1 has a one in seventeen risk.
- The child of a woman with type 1 who gave birth to this child before age twenty-five has a one in twenty-five risk, but if the child was born after the mother turned twenty-five his or her risk is one in one hundred.
- The child's risk doubles if the parent's diabetes was diagnosed before age eleven.
- If both parents have type 1 diabetes, the child's risk jumps to between one in ten and one in four. In addition, most Caucasians with type 1 have genes called *HLA-DR3 or HLA-DR4*. If the parent and child are White and share these genes, the child is at higher risk for developing type 1. Similarly, the HLA-DR7 gene increases the risk of African Americans, and the HLA-BR9 gene increases the risk of Japanese.
- High levels of antibodies against insulin, against the islet cells in the pancreas, or to an enzyme called *glutamicacid decarboxylase*, indicate that a child has a higher risk of developing type 1 diabetes.

What about your child's risk of developing type 2 diabetes?

- Type 2 runs in families because children are taught poor eating habits and nonexercising behaviors from parents.
- Your child's risk for type 2 is one in seven if you were diagnosed with type 2 before the age of fifty. It drops to one in thirteen if you were diagnosed after age fifty.
- Your child's risk is greater if the mother has type 2. If both mother and father have type 2, the risk for the child is one in two.

A risk factor does not mean a certainty. Remember that environmental factors must also exist. So, get your kids eating a healthy diet and move more by playing active games, with you leading the way, for a win-win situation. For more on the genetics of diabetes see the National Institutes of Health's *The Genetic Landscape of Diabetes* (http://www.ncbi.nlm.nih.gov/bookshelf/br.fcgi?book=diabetes), a free online book for people interested in learning more.

New Developments on the Horizon

The cure for diabetes may be closer than you think. The following are some types of research that may provide answers to better control and perhaps prevention.

- ✓ A vaccine to prevent type 1 diabetes.
  Stage of development: The vaccine, named Diamyd and produced by Diamyd Medical, is in Phase III trials (for descriptions of the various phases of drug trials, see Chapter 4).
- ✓ A medication that alters the genes believed to cause insulin resistance in people with type 2 diabetes.
  Stage of development: Currently known as MBX-102, Johnson & Johnson's drug is undergoing Phase II clinical trials.
- ✓ Several groups of researchers are studying rare variations in a single gene that can lead to a wide variety of autoimmune disorders. The gene encodes an enzyme protein called *sialic acid acetylesterase*, or SIAE. This enzyme regulates

What Nurses Know...

If you do any research on the Internet, add the current year after your search term to get the latest posting listed first. There is at lot of outdated and misleading information on the Web, so at least you will eliminate the old news items. As for the misleading ones, compare several current listings to eliminate the odd, different, or contrary postings that may only be someone's opinion and not from a credible source. Check the list of credible sources in the Resources section at the back of this book.

the activity of the immune system's antibody-producing B cells. About two to three percent of people with autoimmune disorders have defects in the enzyme that allow B cells to run amok and make antibodies that attack the body. The hope is that a treatment can be developed to stop this from happening.

Because what we don't know about our health can and does cause damage to glucose-sensitive organs, the diagnosis of anyone at risk for diabetes and treatment at the earliest possible opportunity are critical.

A diagnosis of diabetes can be very overwhelming and frightening. I hope that, with the information on various treatment options available today, living within the guidelines of a healthy lifestyle as outlined in the following chapters will be as doable for you as it has become for me. No one is perfect, but the goal of being healthy and living a healthy life should be important for everyone, not just those of us with diabetes.

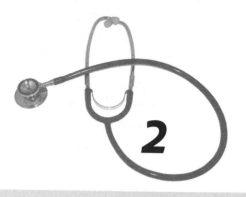

2

What Can I Eat?

After the doctor told me I had diabetes, I was in shock. All I could think about was that it was 3 PM and I had no idea what I could eat or should cook for dinner.   RITA

The American Diabetes Association (ADA) states that the goals of treatment for diabetes are to prevent or delay long-term complications while minimizing the occurrence of low blood sugar. Nutrition, exercise, and medication (when needed) are the cornerstones of successfully treating all classifications of diabetes. In addition to diet and physical activity there are lifestyle modifications, which include smoking cessation and normalization of blood pressure and blood cholesterol.

Early on in my career as a diabetic, a very wise physician said to me "Diabetics have to do what everyone else ought to do." It changed my life and my attitude toward myself and toward the disease itself. As I worked on controlling my blood sugar by eating wisely, exercising, and taking multiple injections of insulin, I felt superior to my peers instead of feeling sorry for myself. I then felt I was choosing to live a healthy lifestyle instead of being forced into it. Sometimes bad things can have good consequences.

Nutrition

Diet is simply what we eat: good, bad or indifferent. We can have a healthy or unhealthy diet. The word *diet* by itself has no negative connotations except those we choose to give it. It can be high fat, high carbohydrate, high fast food, high junk food, high calorie, or restrictive in terms of all of the above, or it can be so low in calories as to deprive our body of the nutrients to sustain life. So, focusing on nutrition and avoiding the negative images the word *diet* has come to evoke may improve your attitude and motivate you to make healthier food choices. In the rest of this chapter I cover the basics of nutrition, weight loss and its ramifications for those of us with diabetes, carbohydrate counting, and what to eat when you are sick.

First let me say that a nutrition plan of action must take into consideration culture, lifestyle, finances, and your readiness to learn and change. You have already shown you are ready by getting this book and reading this chapter, so let's begin.

The basic elements of a diet include carbohydrates, protein, fats, vitamins, minerals, and water. Of these six nutrients the only ones that provide calories are carbohydrates and protein, which have four calories per gram, and fat, which yields a whopping nine calories per gram. Anyone who wants to lose weight must definitely be concerned about how much fat he or she consumes.

CARBOHYDRATES
Blood sugar is influenced by the amount and type of carbohydrates consumed and whether protein and fat are eaten along with it. For instance, an orange is metabolized more slowly than orange juice and takes longer to increase blood sugar. An orange

eaten after cereal and milk or eggs and sausage takes even longer to metabolize. Protein and fat eaten with carbohydrate-containing foods slow down its absorption and thus the resulting blood sugar rise.

Dietary carbohydrate is the major contributor to blood glucose concentration after a meal. It is an important source of energy; water-soluble vitamins, such as the B complex and vitamin C; minerals; and fiber. Because almost all carbohydrates one eats (except for fiber) are absorbed into the blood as glucose, the recommended range of carbohydrate intake is forty-five to sixty-five percent of the total calories. In addition, because the brain and central nervous system can use only glucose as an energy source, restricting one's total carbohydrate intake to <130 g/day is a bad idea. Carbohydrates come from fruit (fructose); milk (lactose); grains, such as bread and cereal; starches, such as pasta and rice; starchy vegetables (corn, peas, and all kinds of beans); and table sugar (sucrose). Yes, people with diabetes can eat sugar. The body metabolizes sugar as a carbohydrate. However, all carbs are not created equal. The empty carbohydrate calories in regular sodas and sugary desserts and snacks contain no nutritive value and should be limited. In addition, desserts and snacks with sugar or high-fructose corn syrup also usually have a high fat content, contributing to increased calories and weight gain.

If you take insulin, you should try to match the number of carbohydrates in a meal or snack with the appropriate amount of insulin (see Chapter 4). Fiber is a complex carbohydrate that does not get absorbed in the body, so technically it should be subtracted from the total carb grams. The recommended amount of fiber per day should equal twenty to thirty-five grams. Fiber increases the speed with which food travels through the digestive system; helps to retain bulk and water in the stool as it enters the rectum; and stimulates the urge to defecate, thus preventing constipation. Fiber fills you up, so you eat less. It is also a magnet for cholesterol and carries it out of the body, lowering low-density lipoproteins (the "bad" cholesterol). Fiber-rich foods include oats; wheat bran; fresh fruit with edible skin;

and fresh vegetables, which can be consumed separately or in a salad. When buying cereal or bread, look for those labeled *whole wheat*, not just *wheat* or *100% wheat*, and *whole multigrain*, not just *twelve-grain, fifteen-grain*, or *multigrain*. If you are not used to eating fiber-rich foods, start slowly or you may feel gassy and bloated. You also need six to eight glasses of noncarbonated liquid to help flush the fiber out of your body.

NATURAL VERSUS ARTIFICIAL SWEETENERS

Table sugar (sucrose) is a natural sweetener. So are honey, molasses, and high-fructose corn syrup. All have empty calories and carbs but can be consumed by persons with diabetes in moderation. Another natural sweetener comes from the stevia plant. In December 2008, the Food and Drug Administration (FDA) gave a "generally recognized as safe" status to Truvia and PureVia, both of which are wholly derived from the stevia plant and have no calories. Since then, combinations have come on the market, such as Only Sweet, a combination of maltodextrine and stevia, also with zero calories, and Sun Crystals, a combination of Truvia and pure cane sugar that has five calories per packet. With obesity and diabetes on the rise, other products are sure to follow. All of these preparations can be found in regular grocery stores and are safe in moderation for nonpregnant adults.

What about artificial sweeteners? The newest one that I am aware of has been on the market since its FDA approval in 1998. It is the yellow packet, sucralose, with the trade name Splenda (and many chain store equivalents). It has been deemed safe by many studies and by the FDA. It is 600 times sweeter than sugar, and it can be used in baking and at high heat levels. Although it is made from chemically altered sugar, it is not absorbed by the body and thus has no calories. To increase fiber in the diet, 1 g of fiber is added to specially marked packets of Splenda, which increases the carbs to two grams per packet but still zero calories. Splenda is also marketed as a sugar blend and a brown sugar blend for baking. These blends decrease the sugar needed in baked goods by half but still have ten calories and two grams of carbs per half-teaspoon. If you want to eat something made with these Splenda blends and you need the carb information to decide on an insulin dose, ask how much of this blend was used and divide by the number of servings per cake, pie, or cookie. If it is more than half a teaspoon, cut your serving to this amount. Multiply the number of half-teaspoons of your serving size by ten calories and two grams of carbs, or use the nutrition facts listed in the recipe. Even though the sugar is decreased, baked goods provide calories and carbs that must be counted.

Two other commonly used artificial sweeteners are aspartame (Equal; NutraSweet; and other generic names), in the blue packets, and saccharin (Sweet & Low and other generic names), in the pink packets. Both are unstable at high temperatures and are safe in moderate amounts. However, many object to the taste or bitter aftertaste (saccharin), and others react with headaches (aspartame) or fear the old studies in animals that linked saccharine in large amounts with cancer. Another artificial sweetener is sodium cyclamate, which was banned in the United States in 1969 but can still be found in other countries.

I need to say a word about sugar-free candy, gum, chocolate, and other products. They are often sweetened with *sugar alcohol*, which is listed on the nutrition facts label under "total carbohydrates" if present. The list includes mannitol, sorbitol, xylitol, maltitol, and other *itol* sweeteners. They do contribute to blood sugar but are slowly absorbed. They also stimulate the bowels, and even a listed serving size may cause cramps and diarrhea in some people. I discuss chocolate further in the section labeled "Fats."

Until I was diagnosed with diabetes, I used to hate the words "in moderation." What does it really mean? The meaning becomes clear when you monitor your blood sugar and your weight to see how consuming these products affect your body, from no effect to greatly increasing your blood glucose levels and weight gain. When considering whether a sweetener is safe, remember that if sugar, or any other carbohydrate source, raises blood glucose to an unhealthy level, glucose-sensitive organs, such as the eyes,

What Nurses Know...

Nutrient-dense foods provide a high dose of vitamins and minerals for a low calorie count.

kidneys, heart, blood vessels, and nerve endings, can be affected. The bottom line is that sugar or its substitutes can be used in small amounts to enhance your enjoyment of foods. However, you may want to consider choosing more nutrient-dense foods, such as fresh or frozen unsweetened fruit and nonfat yogurt, to satisfy your sweet tooth, with a small serving of low-caloric sweet treats on occasion.

PROTEIN

Protein is need to build and repair cells and body tissue as well as to enhance our immune system's response to germs, to maintain fluid and electrolyte and acid–base balance, to produce hemoglobin in red cells, and to build or maintain muscle mass. The ADA recommends that low-fat protein comprise ten to thirty-five percent of the calories we eat. Items such as lean meat, chicken, turkey, ham, or fish, as well as low- or no-fat dairy products, should be eaten every day. If you are a vegetarian, substituting vegetable protein from a variety of sources, such as whole grains, legumes (e.g., beans), vegetables, and starches, as well as eggs and low-fat dairy products, to meet your protein needs will also increase your carbohydrate intake, so they need to be counted carefully, especially if you are giving yourself insulin or are taking a medication that increases your own insulin production. For vegans, who eat no animal products, meeting calcium, iron, and vitamin B-12 needs can be difficult, and they may need to supplement their diets with a multivitamin and mineral source. Calcium, which is needed for strong teeth and bones, is found not only in dairy products such as milk, cheese, and yogurt but also in soy products, such as soy milk, soy yogurt, and tofu, as well as green leafy vegetables and legumes such as beans and peas in lesser amounts. Iron is part of the hemoglobin molecule in red cells and thus is needed for the transport of oxygen to all of the cells of the body. The iron in vegetables and legumes is much harder to digest and absorb than that in egg yolks and red meat, so eating more vegetables containing iron or taking an iron supplement may be necessary. Vitamin B-12, which is needed for red blood cell production, is found naturally only in animal products. There are pastas and other vegan foods fortified with this essential nutrient, but you have to look for them. There are so many good, low-calorie protein choices that, unless a person is sick or unable to consume them, artificially or supplemental protein sources are unnecessary, expensive, and probably unwise.

FATS

Fats are a very important part of our diet. They help the absorption of fat-soluble vitamins and provide essential fatty acids (which the body needs but cannot manufacture). They provide concentrated stored energy and fuel muscle movement. Fat cells pad internal organs and insulate the body against temperature extremes. They also form the major component of cell walls and are the raw material from which hormones, enzymes, bile, and vitamin D are made. Fats also stimulate appetite, make meats tender, and contribute to the feeling of fullness. The problem is that they provide nine calories per gram and contribute to weight gain more than any other nutrient. But let's look at the good, the bad, and the ugly fats. The American Heart Association and the American Cancer Society, as well as the ADA (2010), recommend that fat should be limited to twenty-five to thirty-five percent of calories per day and that no more than seven percent should come from the saturated fat of animal products, such as meat, poultry, fish, and full-fat dairy products. Trans fatty acids in any oils that are hydrogenated or partially hydrogenated should be avoided altogether. Saturated (the bad) fats and trans (the ugly) fats contribute to total cholesterol and triglycerides in the body and eventually to heart disease; atherosclerosis; high blood pressure; and stroke, as well as some cancers, such as breast and colon cancers. Most fat should come from polyunsaturated (the good) sources, such as vegetable oil and fish oil, and monounsaturated (better) sources, such as canola oil, olive oil, nuts, and avocadoes. Ten percent or more of calories should come from monounsaturated sources. Revised 2006 guidelines for nutritional labels state that manufacturers should list the kinds of fats in each product; however, if the amount of anything, including trans fats, is 0.5 mg or less per serving, the manufacturer can list it as zero. If a person chooses to have more than one serving of the product, the trans fats and other ingredients could add up. If the words *hydrogenated* or *partially hydrogenated* are included anywhere in the list of ingredients, trans fat is present.

Elsewhere in this chapter I recommend fresh vegetable salads as a way to lose weight, fill up, and to take advantage of their high fiber and nutrient content. However, you can turn a wonderful salad into a high-calorie, high-fat meal or side dish by dousing it with a high-fat creamy or oily dressing. Look for light, fat-free, low-calorie bottled dressing at the grocery store and ask for the same at restaurants, then request that it come on the side. You will use much less dressing than the server will put on your salad if the dressing comes separately. Another source of high saturated fat is butter, made from the cream of cow's milk and thus 100% saturated fat. Stick margarine is no better because it is hydrogenated oil and so contains a lot of trans fats and has the same number of calories per serving as butter. Better choices include spreads in tubs (read labels for the lowest amount of saturated and trans fats) and butter sprays. Also, you will use a lot less of the product than you would if you purchased a spread in stick form.

NATURAL VERSUS ARTIFICIAL FAT PRODUCTS

Natural fats come from animal products, such as butter, margarine, mayonnaise, cream, and cheese, as well as vegetable sources, such as nuts, nut butters (e.g., peanut butter), and chocolate. Butter and margarine contain one hundred calories per one-tablespoon serving size, mostly from the eleven fat grams they contain, seven of which are saturated. In addition, most brands of stick margarine contain hydrogenated oil, which contains trans fats, so margarine is actually not healthier than butter. One tablespoon of full-fat mayonnaise, which is made from egg yolks, contains eighty calories and nine grams of fat; the same serving size of light mayonnaise has half the calories and half the fat, most of which is unsaturated and is a rich source of omega-3 fatty acids. If you use mayonnaise, try the light version. You might like it. Full-fat dairy products, including cream, cheese, whole milk, and yogurt, contain saturated fat and thus should be limited, especially if you are trying to lose weight or are at high risk for heart disease. Fortunately, they all come in lighter versions that greatly reduce, or eliminate, the fat content. For example, the only differences among whole milk, 2% milk, and nonfat (skim) milk are the amounts of fat and thus calories. All milk has the same carbohydrate, calcium, and protein content. Try mixing 2% and skim milk or looking for 1% milk if you don't want to drink skim milk. The same goes for yogurt, but fat-free yogurt with more than one hundred calories and twenty grams of carbs per six-ounce cup probably has a syrupy fruit mixture that will increase the carb content and raise your blood sugar. Try making your own by adding cut-up fresh fruit to plain fat-free yogurt and add artificial sweetener if needed. Reduced-fat cheese will decrease the calories but not the protein, calcium, or the taste. Fat-free cheese, on the other hand, tastes like plastic, at least to me.

Nuts and nut butters like peanut butter contain one hundred ninety to two hundred calories; sixteen to seventeen grams of fat, most unsaturated; six to seven grams of carbs; and seven to nine grams of protein per serving. They comprise some of the good fats because they are unsaturated and a good source of protein and omega-3 fatty acids. However, stick to the serving size (one quarter cup of nuts and two tablespoons of nut butters) or weight gain due to their high calorie count is a distinct possibility.

Oils are another source of fat calories, so a little goes a long way. Avoid frying your foods, because even canola or olive oil will be absorbed by the chicken, fish, or vegetable being fried and increase the calorie content of foods no matter what the label states. Choose to "oven fry," bake, or stir-fry foods using olive oil or canola oil in a spritzer to decrease the amount.

Now we come to my favorite indulgence: chocolate. I was once told I could not have chocolate any more. I said I would find a way to keep it in my diet, and I did. Current research has proven that a small amount of dark chocolate, my personal favorite, eaten every day, is heart healthy because it is rich in flavanoids and antioxidants. It relaxes blood vessels, thus decreasing blood pressure; improves mood; and puts a smile on your face—at least, on my face. I did, at one point, make my own chocolate candy to reduce the sugar content without resorting to sugar alcohols in the sugar-free chocolate. Here it is:

A CHOCOLATE-LOVER'S RECIPE FOR LOW-SUGAR CHOCOLATE

2 packets of premelted unsweetened chocolate
1 oz of chocolate chips (about 65 chips or 2 tbsp)
10 packets of Splenda or to taste
1 oz shredded unsweetened coconut
2 tbsp raisins
75 small paper muffin cups

Melt first two ingredients in a double boiler, stirring often. When melted, take off heat. Stir in packets of Splenda and mix thoroughly. Add coconut and raisins and coat with chocolate mixture. Spoon mixture into small paper muffin cups and refrigerate until set.

Nutrition information: per serving size of five small muffins. Calories: 52, 7.5% from fat; fat: 3.9 g, carbs: 4.8 g, fiber: 1.15 g, protein: 0.6 g.

Feel free to make your own alterations to the recipe. Pure, unsweetened cocoa powder has almost no fat or carbohydrates. Unsweetened baking chocolate does have cocoa butter and thus fat calories. According to the FDA, semisweet or dark chocolate must have at least thirty-five percent chocolate liquor (nonalcohol) as well as cocoa butter and sugar. Dark chocolate can have as much as ninety percent chocolate liquor, which replaces most of the cocoa butter and sugar. I find that if it contains over sixty to seventy percent chocolate liquor it is pasty and tastes bitter. Milk chocolate, on the other hand, only has ten to fifteen percent chocolate liquor and more cocoa butter, sugar, and milk or cream. White chocolate has no chocolate liquor. None of the chocolate preparations, including the sugar-free variety, are a low-calorie food if they contain fat. But an ounce serving size of dark chocolate is well worth the calories in my book.

The only artificial fat or fat substitute is olestra, brand name Olean. It is a synthetic oil that is not absorbed by the gut, so there are no fat calories. Snacks made with this substance do taste like the full-fat variety; however, this compound takes fat-soluble vitamins, such as A, D, E, and K, as well as carotinoids (precursors to vitamin A) out of the body as well. Because this fat substitute exits the body in the stool, many people experience cramps, diarrhea, or oily brown staining on underpants, especially if the serving size is exceeded. Procter & Gamble received FDA approval to use olestra as a food additive in 1996. You may remember the controversy surrounding olestra-containing WOW! potato chips, manufactured a few years ago by the Frito-Lay corporation, which was required to note on the product label the fact that it contained olestra as well as a list of possible side effects. The FDA-mandated list of the preceding side effects was removed in 2003, but the negative publicity remained. WOW! chips were taken off the market, but Frito-Lay continues to use olestra in their "light" potato chips, Ruffles, Doritos, Tostitos and other snack foods. Pringles "light" potato chips, all flavors, also contain olestra. They all state "made with olestra" on the front of the package, and Olean or olestra is the second listed ingredient after potatoes. Olestra is *not* in the reduced-fat or baked chips of any manufacturer. Olean may also be found in other "light" or fat-free baked goods, frozen desserts, and snack foods. If you choose to eat these products, stick to the serving size at the top of the nutrition facts label. Always check the ingredients label for Olean or olestra, and avoid these products if you experience gastrointestinal repercussions. If it sounds and tastes too good to be true, it just might be. As another alternative to full-fat snacks, try "baked" products and pretzels, but compare the carb content with the real thing. When manufacturers take out fat, which has nine calories per gram, they may replace it with carbohydrates or protein, which have four calories per gram. The extra protein will not increase blood sugar, but the increased carbs will. Snacking on fresh fruit and veggies is a healthier plan. I have included a recipe for a low-calorie, nonfat, low-carb dip for vegetables.

LOW-CALORIE, NONFAT, LOW-CARB VEGGIE DIP

1 package Ranch dip (or other powdered flavor)
1 pint (16 oz) fat-free sour cream

Mix thoroughly and refrigerate for at least 1 hour.

Nutrition information: per each 2-tbsp serving size.
Calories: 35, fat: 0 g, sodium: 265 mg, total carbohydrates: 6 g, protein: 1 g.

You can use this or a low-calorie, low- or nonfat salad dressing to increase your willingness to eat veggies as a snack. Here are other snack suggestions:

LOW-CARB, HIGH-PROTEIN SNACKS

	Snack	Calories	Carbs	Fiber	Protein
1.	One small unpeeled apple &	63	16 g	3 g	0
	2 tbsp peanut butter	190	7 g	3 g	9 g
2.	Seven reduced-fat Triscuits &	120	23 g	3 g	3 g
	2 wedges light Laughing Cow cheese	70	1 g	0	5 g

(*Continued*)

LOW-CARB, HIGH-PROTEIN SNACKS (Continued)

	Snack	Calories	Carbs	Fiber	Protein
3.	One stick light string cheese &	80	<1 g	0	7 g
	18 all-bran crackers	120	19 g	5 g	3 g
4.	Two 100% whole grain Fig Newtons	110	22 g	2 g	1 g
	& 1/2 cup skim milk	40	6 g	0	4g
5.	One hard-boiled egg &	80	1 g	0	7g
	1 slice double-fiber whole wheat bread	50	13 g	5 g	3 g
6.	Ten baby carrots, 1 cup celery stalks,	52	12 g	2 g	1 g
	& 4 tbsp nonfat ranch dip (see recipe)	60	12 g	0	4 g
7.	One-half cup fat-free cotta ge cheese &	80	8 g	0	12 g
	1/2 cup fresh or frozen blueberries	56	14 g	3 g	1 g
8.	One Fiber One bar &	140	29 g	9 g	2 g
	1/2 cup skim milk	40	6 g	0	4 g
9.	One oz high-fiber cereal &	80	23 g	10 g	4 g
	1/2 cup skim milk	40	6 g	0	4 g
10.	Two oat bran cookies &	26	6 g	0	2 g
	1/2 cup low-fat, no sugar added ice cream	20	22 g	0	3 g
11.	Smoothie: 1 cup skim milk;	80	12 g	0	8 g
	1 cup frozen, unsweetened strawberries; &	77	20 g	5 g	1 g
	artificial sweetener to taste	0	0	0	0
12.	Two light Babybel semisoft cheeses	100	0	0	6 g
13.	Two stalks of celery &	20	4 g	2 g	0
	1 Tbsp peanut butter	95	7 g	3 g	9 g
14.	One-half cup sugar-free pudding	60	13 g	1 g	2 g
15.	Two cups popcorn,	100	12 g	2 g	2 g
	10 sprays of spray butter	0	0	0	0
16.	6 oz light yogurt	90	15 g	0	8 g
17.	Two 1-oz containers sugar-free gelatin	20	0 g	0	2 g
	2 Tbsp light whipped topping	16	2 g	0	0

In the next table I have listed the recommended percentages and what they mean in terms of the range of grams for each nutrient based on the number of calories per day. If you enjoy crunching the numbers as I do, you can individualize this table by following the formula underneath.

GRAMS OF CARBS, PROTEIN, AND FAT

Calories (cal)/day	Carbs (4 cal) 45%–65% of cal	Protein (4 cal) 10%–35% of cal	Fat (9 cal) 25%–35% of cal
1,200	135–195 g	30–105 g	33–47 g
1,500	169–244 g	37.5–131 g	42–58 g
1,800	202.5–292.5 g	45–157.5 g	50–70 g
2,000	225–325 g	50–175 g	55.5–78 g
2,200	247.5–357.5 g	55–192.5 g	61–85.5 g
2,500	281–406 g	62.5–219 g	69.5–97 g
3,000	337.5–487.5 g	75–262.5 g	83–117 g

Calories × percent changed to decimal = cal for nutrient
   cal from nutrient ÷ 4 or 9 = Number of grams
Examples:

$$1,200 \text{ cal} \times 0.45 = 540 \text{ calories for carbs}$$
$$540 \text{ cal} \div 4 \text{ cal/g} = 135 \text{ g}$$
$$1,200 \text{ cal} \times 0.65 = 780 \text{ calories for carbs}$$
$$780 \text{ cal} \div 4 \text{ cal/g} = 195 \text{ g}$$

EXAMPLE BREAKDOWN OF A 1,200 CALORIE WEIGHT LOSS DIET

Meal	Carbs: 45%	Protein: 30%	Fat: 25%
Breakfast	40 g	15 g	10 g
Snack	10 g	10 g	0 g
Lunch	30 g	20 g	10 g
Snack	15 g	0 g	0 g
Dinner	30 g	30 g	10 g
Snack	15 g	15 g	3 g
Dietary total	135 g	90 g	33 g

Nutrition Labels

To figure out the percentage of carbohydrates, protein, and fat you consume, you need to know how to read a nutrition label. If you are not familiar with nutrition labels, it would be helpful at this time to get a package, can, or bread wrapper and follow along while I explain what it contains. The most important thing to look at is the serving size, which is right under the words *Nutrition Facts* at the top. It can be listed as the number of slices; the size of the slice in ounces; the number of cups, from one-quarter of a cup or more; or some other measurable amount (e.g., number of crackers). In the beginning, and periodically throughout your adventure in healthy eating, you will need to use your measuring cups and spoons to get accurate serving sizes. Put what you measure (the serving size) onto a plate you typically use for this food. Notice how much of the plate it covers. After awhile, you may be able to estimate the proper serving size. I still measure cereal and milk because I am tempted to pour more than the correct serving size, and they both contain carbs. It is also helpful to note how many servings a package contains. You might be shocked, for example, to learn that most macaroni and cheese boxes contain four servings, especially if you have been splitting it with one other person (or eating all of it yourself). Once you understand the serving size, realize that every number or percentage listed below it refers to that exact amount. That means if you are eating twice the serving size, you must multiply all the numbers on the nutrition facts label by two, and so on.

Next, look at calories per serving and the number of calories from fat. Divide this number by the total calories to get the percentage of fat per serving. Aim for thirty percent (0.3) or less. The FDA considers a food that contains fewer than one hundred total calories per serving as low calorie, one hundred to three hundred ninety-nine calories as having a moderate amount of calories, and more than four hundred calories as a high calorie food. Next, look at fat and protein grams. Unless you are trying to gain weight, the lower the fat grams, and the higher the protein grams, the better. If you are counting carbs, the total carbohydrate grams is important, not just the grams of sugar, which is included in that total. I have already discussed the importance of fiber; look for at least five grams of fiber per serving of cereal and two and a half to three grams per slice of bread. Compare labels and buy the better source of fiber that tastes good to you and your family.

The last items you should look at on the label are sodium and potassium. Both relate to blood pressure, which can be a problem with anyone who has diabetes. Sodium contributes to raising blood pressure, and potassium helps lower it. It is estimated that the average American consumes about 3,000 mg of sodium per day. We all need sodium in our body to maintain the appropriate concentration of blood and for electrolyte balance; however, the daily sodium intake for healthy people should be about the equivalent of a teaspoon of table salt, or 2,300 mg. If you are already concerned about your blood pressure or are on medication to lower it, a low-sodium diet (2,300 mg) is a must. Stick to fresh or frozen fruit (no sugar added); and fresh or frozen vegetables (not in butter sauce); and limit canned products, deli meats, or processed foods.

According to the April 2010 issue of *Consumer Reports On Health*, 77% of our salt intake comes from packaged and restaurant foods. If you don't prepare your own spaghetti sauce, check and compare jars to find the lowest sodium content per serving. You can easily consume half or more of your 2,300 mg per day with just a one-half cup serving size of this product. Just like getting used to a low-fat diet, a low-sodium diet takes time. Reduce

What Nurses Know...

If you use canned vegetables, rinse the contents thoroughly, and don't use the liquid, to reduce the sodium. Rinsing canned beans also reduces the potential for intestinal gas.

sodium gradually. Start by putting the salt shaker in a cabinet so you have to get up to get it. Replace salt with pepper, the available blends of herbs and spices (e.g., Mrs. Dash), and/or Morton's Lite Salt (a mixture of sodium and potassium chloride). Limit salty snacks like potato chips and pretzels and, when you do have them, stick to the serving size. Potassium also helps with fluid and electrolyte balance as well as nerve stimulation of muscles, including heart muscle. Most potassium is found in cells, but the small amount in blood is critical in maintaining heart rhythm and kidney function. Increasing potassium in your diet is as simple as eating fresh fruit, such as bananas, cantaloupe, and citrus fruit, and vegetables, such as carrots, tomatoes, winter squash, and potatoes. Go to www.dashdiet.org for more information on the DASH diet (Dietary Alternative to Stop Hypertension), which is low in sodium and high in potassium. It includes fresh fruit, vegetables, and whole-grain products. The following are examples of foods that lower blood pressure:

Fiber-Rich Foods
Whole-grain foods
- Brown rice
- Whole wheat bread
- High-fiber cereals

Fruit with edible peel or seeds
- Pears
- Apples
- Berries
- Figs, prunes

Vegetables
- Artichokes
- Celery
- Legumes
- Broccoli
- Peas

Potassium-Rich Foods
- Salt substitutes (100% potassium chloride)
- Light salt (half potassium chloride, half sodium chloride)
- Fresh fruits and vegetables

What Nurses Know...

When your potassium levels are too low you may experience leg and arm muscle cramps, nausea, vomiting, weakness, fatigue, heart palpitations, and abdominal cramps, bloating, or constipation.

Because reading labels can be time consuming at first, start by looking at the products you already have in your refrigerator or pantry. On your next grocery shopping excursion, start with bread or cereal if you find that the products you have been buying are high in calories and fat and low in fiber. Next, look at milk and other dairy products. Look for low-calorie, lowfat milk and yogurt choices. Reduced-fat cheese adds calories, protein, and calcium to your meal without carbs.

Weight Loss

Weight loss is recommended for anyone whose body mass index (BMI) indicates that they are overweight or obese or whose waist measurement is more than forty inches for men and more than thirty-five inches for women.

BODY MASS INDEX

BMI is body weight in kilograms divided by height in meters squared. To calculate BMI using pounds and inches, follow these steps:

1. Multiply weight in pounds by 703.
2. Multiply height in inches times itself.
3. Divide the results of Step 1 by Step 2 and compare with results below.

Example:

1. 170 pounds × 703 = 119,510.
2. 5 feet, 4 inches = 64 × 64 = 4,096
3. 119,510 ÷ 4096 = 29.177 = overweight (see below)

DISEASE RISK BASED ON BODY MASS INDEX (BMI) AND WAIST CIRCUMFERENCE

Weight Category	BMI	Waist Circumference (inches)	
		≤ 40 in men ≤ 35 in women	> 40 in men > 35 in women
Underweight	<18.5	Low	—
Normal weight	18.5–24.9	Low	—
Overweight	25–29.9	Increased	High
Obese	30–39.9	High	Very high
Morbidly obese	≥40	Very high	Extremely high

With permission from Mertig, RG, *The Nurse's Guide to Teaching Diabetes Self-Management*, Springer Publishing Company, LLC, New York, NY.

You can also use the online calculator at www.nhlbisupport.com/bmi/bmicalc.htm

Even a small weight loss of ten to twenty pounds can reverse insulin resistance and improve blood sugar levels. Weight loss should be achieved over a period of time with a loss of one to two pounds per week (more if you are extremely overweight). This can be achieved by portion control, decreasing intake of high-calorie foods and foods with empty calories, and increasing physical activity. The number of calories eaten must not be greater than the number of calories burned, or weight gain will result. Some weight loss diets advertise a weight loss of ten or more pounds per week. That is possible only because this diet causes water loss and puts you at risk for dehydration. Eating at least ten grams of protein at every meal helps to prevent the burning of lean muscle mass when trying to lose weight. Muscles burn more calories even at rest, so maintaining or increasing muscle mass is helpful in losing weight and maintaining that loss.

What Nurses Know . . .

Secretes to Weight Loss

- *Get accurate measuring cups and spoons.*
- *Use smaller plates and bowls.*
- *Divide your plate in half and fill with nonstarchy fresh or cooked vegetables. On the other half put a protein source and a starch.*
- *Substitute herbs and herb blends like Mrs. Dash for salt.*
- *Reduce sugar by one half to three fourths, and double the amount of spices in recipes.*
- *Replace half the fat in baked goods with unsweetened applesauce.*
- *Steam mixed veggies like broccoli, cauliflower, and carrots and top with reduced-fat cheese crumbles, or spritz with spray butter.*
- *Roast vegetables like squash, sweet potato, or colorful peppers to enhance their sweetness.*
- *Don't skip meals or go hungry. Snack on fresh fruit and veggies.*
- *Drink cold water or unsweetened, decaffeinated iced tea before meals and snacks. You'll burn calories heating it to body temperature and will partially fill your stomach.*
- *Brush your teeth and/or chew sugarless gum after dinner to curb evening snacking.*
- *Weigh yourself often: every day or every week to test out one or more strategies, for a pat on the back, or to get back on track.*
- *Stop wolfing down meals and snacks. Set a timer for at least twenty minutes, and enjoy the food until the timer rings. This will help you slow down your eating habits and give your body time to register fullness.*

The ADA recommends that caloric intake for most adults should not be less than 1,000-1,200 Kcal/day for women and 1,200-1,600 Kcal/day for men. Anything less will result in a reprogramming of the rate at which calories are burned. If our bodies think we are starving, the absorption of nutrients by the small intestine gets very efficient, and our basal metabolic rate decreases to conserve energy. Thus, when we increase calories after losing weight, we gain it right back and even more. It takes much more effort to increase one's metabolic rate to burn more calories than to decrease the rate. Any caloric restriction below the recommended limits just stated will result in what many people call *yo-yo dieting* and is counterproductive.

One of the most useful tools to achieve weight loss is a dietary journal. Keeping track of everything eaten, the timing of meals and snacks, the amounts of each food item consumed (which means measuring and weighing), to accurately calculate calories and grams of carbohydrates, protein, and fat, and to record any emotions that accompany eating patterns is very useful in generating an action plan to change and improve eating habits. Of course, physical activity is a part of any weight loss program. To lose one to two pounds per week, we must decrease current intake by five hundred to one thousand calories per day, or burn that much by increasing physical activity, or a combination of both modalities. Losing weight can be difficult, but a sign I once saw, "Nothing tastes as good as thin feels," always makes me smile when I think about it. More information about weight loss drugs and surgery for obesity can be found at www.weightwatchers. com. Search the site for "The Physics of Weight Loss," then scroll down to and click on "Bariatric Surgery and Weight Loss" and/or "Weight-Loss Medications."

THE SLEEP-WEIGHT CONNECTION

Sleep deprivation is common today, but it can make you sick and fat. Several studies have shown the connection between lack of sufficient sleep and obesity in both adults and children. Inadequate sleep has been linked to lower levels of the hormone leptin, which signals to our brain that we are full. In children, one study showed that inadequate sleep was the biggest contributor to childhood obesity, more so than any other factor. How can you tell how much sleep you need? Because we are all different, a good test is to wake up without an alarm clock. When you wake up this way, your body is telling you that you are rested. If you routinely sleep longer on the weekend, or when you don't have to be somewhere, that should tell you something. On average, most people need between seven and eight hours of sleep every night, although some may wake up after only four or five hours and feel rested, whereas others need ten or more hours. So, one of the most pleasant ways to lose weight is to make sure you get enough sleep.

Food Pyramid Versus the Dietary Guidelines

The old food pyramid did not include physical activity and emphasized starches and protein without sufficient fruit and vegetables. Also, there were no discretionary calories, and it was difficult to individualize a meal plan. The 2005 Dietary Guidelines for Americans developed by the U.S. Department of Agriculture and the U.S. Department of Health and Human Services were an attempt to help people individualize the food pyramid and make it more user friendly. The web site www.mypyramid.gov provides authoritative advice for anyone age two years and older concerning healthy dietary habits that reduce the risk of major chronic diseases. All you have to do is key in your age, gender, and physical activity level—truthfully—and a personalized dietary recommendation based on the new 2010 guidelines is produced. It details the kind and amounts of foods to eat each day and provides encouragement to improve dietary choices and make lifestyle changes in small, incremental steps. "My Pyramid Tracker" provides a means to monitor your progress.

Thankfully, the diabetic (ADA) diets of the past are gone. What we need to remember is that a diet appropriate for someone with diabetes is a nutritious, well-balanced one full of choices, including sugar. It is a diet that meets all of the recommendations from the ADA, the American Heart Association, the American Cancer Society, and the 2010 Dietary Guidelines for Americans. It is full of vitamins, minerals, antioxidants, flavanoids, and other nutrients that we all need to stay healthy. The 2010 Dietary Guidelines were released on June 15, 2010, by the Dietary Guidelines Advisory Committee, which researched and consolidated nutritional data over the last five years. The guidelines focus on the prevention of obesity and chronic disease and advises Americans to do the following:

- Minimize time spent in front of the TV and computer screens.
- Eat more home-cooked meals so you can lower the sodium and trans fat content of the foods you eat.
- Consume more fruits, vegetables, and whole grains, and decreased your consumption of processed foods.
- Minimize consumption of added sugars, as in sweets and regular sodas; refined grains, such as white bread and white rice; and sodium. Avoid adding these at the table, and minimize the amount in cooking.
- Increase physical activity for everyone, not just the overweight. All age brackets benefit from becoming more active. Some physical activity is better than none, and more is better.

To view the full text of the 2010 Dietary Guidelines, go to www. cnpp.usda.gov/dgas2010-dgacreport.htm.

Someone is always telling me that I cannot eat this or that because I have diabetes. My answer to them is usually "If I can't eat it, maybe you shouldn't eat it." I sometimes also add "If I can give myself sufficient insulin to control blood sugar as your pancreas does, all that will happen is that we will both put on weight."

Carbohydrate Counting

If insulin administered to or produced by your body should match the amount of carbohydrates ingested, then counting carbs is a worthwhile endeavor. The foods that have the greatest effect on blood sugar include the items in the bread/cereal/starch food group; the fruit group; the milk group; starchy vegetables such as peas, corn, lima beans, potatoes, and dried or canned beans; and, of course, sweets. The amount of each is also important. The following is a practical guide to counting grams of carbohydrates.

The bread/cereal/starch group equals 15 g of carbs per serving

Bread	1 slice
Pasta	1/2 cup (cooked)
Dry cereal	1 oz (1/4 to 1½ cups based on cereal)
Cooked cereal	1/2 cup
Starchy vegetables	1/3 to 1/2 cup (cooked)
Potato with skins	1/2 potato (2¼ × 4¾), or 1/2 cup slice/mash/canned

The fruit group equals 15 g of carbohydrates per serving

Fresh fruit	1 medium piece or 1/2 grapefruit, 1 cup strawberries, 1/2 cup blueberries, 1/2 banana or 1 small banana
Fruit juice	1/3 to 1/2 cup (2.7-4 oz)
Frozen fruit	See nutrition label for serving size
Canned fruit	See nutrition label for serving size (use only if canned in fruit juice)

The milk group equals 12 g of carbohydrates per serving

Milk	1 cup
Yogurt, plain	3/4 cup or 6 oz

Nonstarchy vegetables have five grams of carbohydrates per half cup cooked or one cup raw. I usually eat as much of this food group as I want to avoid getting hungry. Meats and fats have no carbohydrates unless cooked or mixed with something that does.

According to Warshaw and Boderman in their book *Practical Carbohydrate Counting*, carbohydrates begin to raise blood glucose within fifteen minutes after starting to eat them and are converted

What Nurses Know . . .

Counting carbs has gotten much easier with food labels and their listed nutritional contents. A serving size is identified at the top of the food label. If a serving size is doubled, the carb grams, as well as all other entities on the label, must also be doubled.

to nearly 100% glucose within two hours. Because I have listed serving sizes for whole fruit and fruit juices, I need to differentiate between the two. *Fruit juice* usually has very little fiber and is already in liquid form, so it is absorbed very quickly and raises blood sugar within a few minutes. Juice is ideal for raising blood sugar when you are experiencing hypoglycemia, but otherwise choose the whole fruit or frozen fruit without added sugar. Whole fruit has fiber and its breakdown to a liquid form by the stomach burns calories before it can be absorbed. Blood glucose rises much more slowly when fruit is eaten, especially after a meal. Healthy, low-carb juices to drink include tomato and V8 juices, although they have a moderately high sodium content. See boxes displayed earlier in this chapter for low-carb, high-protein snacks and low-carb beverages. For a list of the lowest carb fruits and vegetables, as well as for other suggestions for snacks, lunch, and dinner ideas, visit www.dlife.com/food.

So, how many carbs should you eat? The following are some suggestions, depending on total calories:

Women: 45-60 g/meal
Men: 60-75 g/meal
Snacks: 15-30 g (up to two snacks as needed)

I have not written about the glycemic index as a way of counting carbs, because I find it cumbersome. It is much easier for me to remember the grams of the various food groups and keep a rough idea of their serving size than to look up every product on the glycemic index. My other objection to using the glycemic index is that some high-fat foods are on the low end of the index because the fat content blunts the blood sugar spike. If you want more information on the glycemic index, go to www.carbs-information.com/glycemic-index-food-chart.htm.

To help put everything in this chapter together, you need to get a food count book that lists calories, carbs, protein, fat, sodium, and fiber. It should include fresh foods as well as brand names. Nutrients of foods from fast food and chain restaurants can be found on their various Web sites. Be prepared with healthy options before you eat out. You can create a personalized menu using foods from the list at www.changing-diabetes-us.com, or go to www.mypyramid.gov for answers to questions, and let this helpful site plan meals for you. It might also be useful to get a cookbook or use recipes that list serving size and nutrient content, especially calories and carb and fiber grams.

If you have been following the debates on healthcare in Washington, you know that it will take awhile to unravel all that is in this massive bill. However, one thing tucked into this bill might be helpful when eating out at fast food and other chain restaurants is a requirement that calorie counts be on menus, menu boards, and even drive-thru boards. The FDA will have a year to write new rules that must be followed by any restaurant that has twenty or more locations. Other nutritional information besides calories will have to be posted somewhere else in the restaurant. The requirements will be enforced by the FDA with possible criminal penalties for noncompliance. This is something to look forward to in 2011.

Alcohol: Pros and Cons

Many people think that anyone with diabetes should not drink alcoholic beverages. Studies have shown that moderate drinking, which means no more than one to two drinks per day, can reduce the risk of heart disease by 30 to 50 percent by increasing high-density lipoprotein ("good" cholesterol) levels and preventing clot formation in the arteries. The Johns Hopkins White Paper *Nutrition and Weight Control for Longevity* (2010) lists the following recommendations with regard to alcohol:

- If you currently don't drink alcohol, do not start.
- If you are a man, limit yourself to one to two drinks per day and cut this in half if you are over the age of 65. It takes longer to detoxify alcohol as we age.
- If you are a woman, limit intake to no more than one drink per day and take half that amount if over 65.
- The type of alcoholic drink does not matter. Wine (red or white), beer, and spirits have the same effect on heart health.
- Heavy alcohol consumption (defined as more than two drinks per day) can cause or worsen high blood pressure, heart disease, stroke, and liver disease.
- Some people should not drink. Anyone with high triglyceride levels, uncontrolled high blood pressure, an inflamed pancreas (pancreatitis), liver disease, or who has had problems with alcohol in the past should not drink. Alcohol can also interfere with many medications, so check with your prescribing healthcare practitioner.
- Do not drink and drive or operate heavy machinery.

Alcohol can be part of the diet for a person with diabetes as long as it is used in moderation and the calories and carbohydrates (if any) are accounted for. Alcohol delivers seven calories per gram and is metabolized like a fat. One drink is defined as a 12-oz beer, 5 oz wine, or 1.5 oz distilled spirits. Beer, sweet wines, and after-dinner liqueurs have carbs that need to be counted. Don't mix alcohol with anything that has carb value, like fruit juices or regular soft drinks, for the same reason. Check out Baja Bob's sugar-free drink mixers at www.bajabob.com if you are looking for some tasty mixers that come in bottles or in single-serving packets. No alcohol is required.

Alcohol can cause hypoglycemia, so it should always be consumed with food. The reason for this is that alcohol is detoxified in the liver. If hypoglycemia occurs, alcohol prevents the liver from responding to glucagon by releasing stored sugar, so one's blood glucose may drop dangerously low. In addition, because the behavior of someone experiencing low blood sugar is often mistaken for drunkenness, a diabetic with alcohol on his or her breath may not be treated appropriately, potentially resulting in brain damage and even death from severe hypoglycemia.

Sick Day Management

This is one of the most important pieces of information for someone with diabetes to know in order to prevent further illness

WHAT TO EAT OR DRINK WHEN YOU'RE SICK: FOODS THAT HAVE 15 GRAMS OF CARBS

Food Item	Amount
Fruit juice	1/2 cup
Fruit-flavored drink (not diet)	1/2 cup
Soda (regular, not diet)	1/2 cup
Jell-O (regular, not sugar-free)	1/2 cup
Popsicle (regular, not sugar-free)	1/2 cup
Sherbet	1/2 cup
Saltine crackers	6 crackers
Bread	1 slice
Milk	1 cup
Soup	1 cup
Ice cream (regular)	1/2 cup
Applesauce	1/2 cup
Pudding (regular)	1/4 cup
Macaroni, noodles, rice	1/3 cup (cooked)
Potatoes, beans, cereal	1/2 cup (cooked)

What Nurses Know...

The following items each equals about 10 to 15 g of carbohydrates

Food Item	Amount
Sugar packets	2 to 3 packets
Fruit juice	1/2 cup (4 oz)
Soda (not diet)	1/2 cup (4 oz)
Hard candy	3 to 5 pieces
Sugar or honey	4 tsp
Glucose tablets	3 to 4 tablets
Glucose gel packets	1 packet

from hypo- or hyperglycemia. Testing blood sugar every two to four hours is a must. If a blood sugar reading is high, you must stay hydrated with diet or noncaloric drinks such as water, broth, sugar-free tea or coffee, and sugar-free gelatin or Popsicles. If a blood sugar reading is normal or low, then regular soda or fruit drinks should be consumed. Start drinking fluids slowly one to two hours after vomiting or diarrhea.

If you have already given yourself insulin or taken a medication that increases your production of insulin, you should have glucose tablets or gels available to prevent or treat a low blood sugar.

Be sure to test first before assuming your blood glucose level will drop. Often an illness or infection will stress the body enough to release hormones that will raise blood sugar.

When you have diabetes, learning about nutrition can be an adventure in good health for the whole family, if it is approached in a positive manner. Since my diagnosis, my family has benefited from a healthy diet because I never prepare anything I should not eat. The emphasis should be on making changes gradually and keeping some favorite foods in the diet for eating on occasion. Remember, there is no bad food, so get rid of the guilt. However, some foods are better for us than others and should become part of our everyday meal plan.

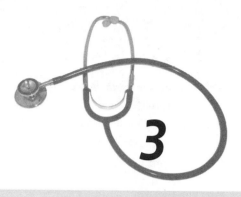

3

Why Should I Exercise?

I am too busy to exercise and I really can't afford to belong to a gym. I just like relaxing in front of the TV.   ANNA

I know I should exercise, but every time I try, my blood sugar drops low and I have to stop. Is it really necessary and, if so, how can I prevent low blood sugar?   JOHN

Have you ever said something like either Anna or John did? Are you still fighting the idea of exercising even though you know you should? I hope that in this chapter I can give you more to think about and help you learn new and different ways to become more physically active. I have decided to use the term *physical activity* interchangeably with *exercise* because, just like the word *diet*, *exercise* has a negative connotation for many people. Exercise seems to portray punishing athletic endeavors, such as long, boring walks; sweaty marathon jogging; or weight lifting at the gym. All *physical activity* means is physical movement, the kind of activity that gets you out of bed in the morning and keeps you moving throughout the day. It is important to remind ourselves that it all counts toward keeping our muscles toned and our bones strong. What we all need is more of it. I was in Chicago visiting my daughter and her family recently and was amazed to see fewer obese children and adults than in my own suburb of Richmond, Virginia. The population in this and, I presume, other large cities is very dense, with most people living in high-rise apartments and condos. Space to park a car is at a premium, and gas prices are terribly high. Most Chicagoans walk to stores, restaurants, friends' homes, and often to work. At the very least, they have to walk to the bus or other mass transit station. Avoiding stairs is often also not an option. During my visit we ate out a lot, so I was shocked when I returned home to find that I had lost weight. What a refreshing turn of events! As a result, I am now walking to the drugstore, library, and anywhere else that is a mile or less away. It saves gas, and I notice more what is going on near where I live. Of course, this is presuming there is no inclement weather, but my experience in Chicago increased the amount of walking I do. It takes a little planning so that I don't just head for the car every time I need to run an errand.

What Counts As Physical Activity

Physical activity is anything that gets your arms and/or legs moving. If you do it for at least twenty minutes and it gets your heart and your lungs working harder, we call it *aerobic exercise*. It conditions both the heart and lungs so they are in better shape to work more efficiently, even at rest. If you work on separate muscle groups, such as the upper arms, thighs, or abdomen, we call it *weight training*, and it is an example of *anaerobic*, or passive, exercise. What about stretching your muscles and increasing flexibility? Yes, that is exercise, too. Isometrics, in which you use your own body to push and pull against something, also is a form of exercise, called *resistance training*. Even relaxation exercises can benefit our muscles and stamina. What about work around the house or in the yard? It all counts and burns calories. The following are some examples:

CALORIES BURNED PER HALF-HOUR OF WORK

Activity	Calories burned
Making the bed	68
Doing laundry	73
Washing dishes	78
Ironing	78
Dusting	85
Cooking	85
Washing the car	102
Washing windows	102
Sweeping	112
Vacuuming	119
Scrubbing floors	129
Gardening	136
Raking	146
Yard work	170
Mowing the lawn	187
Rearranging furniture	204
Shoveling snow	204
Carrying 15 lbs up or down stairs	289

These statistics, from www.caloriesperhour.com, are for a 150-lb, 35-year-old woman doing thirty solid minutes of everyday chores around the house.

Types of Exercise

In case you are wondering exactly what you should do to increase your physical activity level and why, the following discussion should be of interest to you.

AEROBIC EXERCISE

The 2010 Dietary Guidelines for Americans, published by the U.S. Department of Agriculture, state that most people should aim for a minimum of thirty minutes of aerobic exercise per day on most days. Aerobic exercise is defined as any physical activity that increases your heart and respiratory rates and causes you to break a light sweat. This includes walking inside or outside, dancing, using an aerobic DVD, swimming, water aerobics, low-impact aerobics class, ice or roller skating, tennis (even hitting the backboard), biking inside or outside, mowing the lawn, gardening, housework, and so on. Weight-bearing exercises to keep calcium in our bones and prevent osteoporosis consist of all of these except exercises in water, because water exercises, although aerobic, do not put pressure on the long bones of the arms or legs. This is why they are good for those of us with arthritis, but we also need to do some other exercise, such as weight training, to help our bones stay strong.

Children and teens should aim for at least sixty minutes of exercise a day. Some of this time could be during an active gym class or actively playing during recess at school. This never used to be a problem because most kids enjoy being physically active. As long as excessive TV, video, or computer games and other sedentary pursuits don't take over their playtimes, children will be active. With the dangers today of abduction and physical harm comes the problem of trying to keep our children safe by confining them to the house even when we are present. Parents need to find alternatives to the naturally active play that used to be part of growing up. Enrolling children in after-school day care, YMCA programs, or other supervised activities are only a few of the possibilities. Swapping days with a neighbor or friend with a child of similar age, or paying this person to watch your child as well as his or her own, may be feasible. Actively playing with children or grandchildren after work takes thought and creativity but may be the solution to physical inactivity for both the child and the adult. For me, playing ring-around-the-rosy and other games with my almost–three-year-old grandson meet all the criteria for aerobic activity.

In a large study of adults with prediabetes, The Diabetes Prevention Program, which comprises one hundred fifty minutes of physical activity a week, or thirty minutes on five days a week, helped prevent or delay the diagnosis of type 2 diabetes in the study participants. They also lost ten to twenty pounds by eating a healthier diet. If this sounds like too much for you, start slowly, with ten minutes of physical activity, and add five to ten minutes per day every week or so, until you have reached thirty minutes or more. Exercise doesn't even have to be done all at one time. Three ten-minute periods can also be useful.

STRENGTH TRAINING

Increasing muscle tone, strength, and size requires that you lift more weight than you are used to. The more muscle tissue we have, the more calories we burn every hour, day and night. Start with 1- or 2-lb weights in each hand, and slowly do bicep curls. Raise the weights over your head and slowly lower them behind your head and neck to strengthen the triceps. Raise the weights with straight arms to the side to work a combination of muscles, including those in the shoulders. For legs, try hooking your legs under a heavy piece of furniture and, with knees loose, contract your thigh muscles slowly, and try to lift. Hold for a count of ten and then relax slowly. Squats can be done using an exercise ball or beach ball against a wall. With your back on the ball and your feet in front of your body, lean back and lower your body to a sitting position, rolling it against the ball for stability. If your knees go over your toes when bent, move your feet farther away from the wall. Do eight repetitions of each exercise, pause for one minute, and do eight more. Do them slowly, and take deep breaths throughout. When doing two sets becomes easy, either increase the number of repetitions to twelve per set or increase the weights. Remember to move slowly; increase the weights slowly; and, above all, skip a day before exercising the same muscles. It takes thirty-six to forty-eight hours for muscles to rebuild, so alternate days for strength training your arms and legs. The muscles of the abdomen rebuild in twenty-four hours, so abdominal exercises can be done every day.

STRETCHING OR FLEXIBILITY EXERCISES

The movements involved in stretching and flexibility exercises help your joints remain flexible and injury free during any kind of exercise. Joints and muscles need to be warmed up before stretching, so do some jumping jacks, arm movements, and sitting and then standing for a few minutes to get the blood flowing. Then focus on stretching each joint you will use in whatever aerobic activity you have planned.

1. For feet and ankles: Stand on the edge of a stair tread and go up on your tiptoes, then let your heels slowly drop slightly below the tread. Repeat a few times, holding onto the banister or wall.

2. For calves and Achilles tendons: Stand at arm's length from a wall with your palms on the wall and your fingers toward the ceiling. With left knee slightly bent, place your right leg behind, with heel and foot flat on the floor. Bend your left knee until you feel a stretch in the calf and Achilles tendon of the right leg. Hold for ten to thirty seconds. Switch legs and repeat.

3. For thighs: Put one hand on the wall and with the other hand grasp the foot on same side. Pull the heel toward your buttocks and hold for ten to thirty seconds. Feel the stretch in front of your thigh. Switch legs and hands and repeat.

4. For hamstrings (back of thigh): Stand behind a chair far enough away so you can bend at the hips and place your hands with arms straight on back of chair. Feel the stretch in the back of your thigh. Hold for ten to thirty seconds.

5. For hips and lower back: Lie flat on your back. Bend both knees and clasp them with your hands. Pull your knees toward your shoulders as you exhale. Hold for ten to thirty seconds, breathing normally. Feel the stretch in your lower back.

6. For shoulder and upper back: Lie on your back, with your head on a pillow and your legs out straight or with a rolled towel under your knees. With arms at your side, bend your elbow so your fingers point to the ceiling and your palm faces forward. Slowly roll your arms toward the floor until you feel the stretch in your shoulders. Hold for ten to thirty seconds. Raise your forearms slowly off the floor so your hands point to the ceiling, then them return to your side.

7. For sides: Stand or sit and reach upward with one arm and hand while the other reaches down the other side of your body. Hold for ten to thirty seconds. Feel the stretch along the rib cage, back of arm, and waist. Repeat with other side.

8. For triceps: Bend one arm behind your back and hold with your other hand at the elbow. Pull toward the opposite side until you feel the stretch along the back of your upper arm. Hold for ten to thirty seconds and repeat with the other arm.

9. For neck and upper back: Slowly move your chin to your chest and hold, then bend your neck backward and hold. Bend your neck sideways toward each shoulder and hold. Turn head so you are looking over each shoulder in turn and hold.

Repeat these stretches after you exercise. This is probably the most important time to stretch, to prevent the exercised muscles from getting tight.

BALANCE EXERCISES

Aging is the number one reason for poor balance in most people. However, people with diabetes may have a few more issues to contend with, such as neuropathy causing tingling and numbness in feet and uncorrected vision problems, like cataracts and retinopathy. (See Chapter 6 for more about diabetes-related complications.) Poor balance can lead to falls, causing fractures and possibly head injuries. There are many ways to improve balance, including practicing Tai Chi, yoga, and Pilates in addition to walking and general strength training. Practice the following exercises to see how good your sense of balance is. If needed, hold on to a wall or a chair.

- Do heel-to-toe walking (place the heel of one foot in front of and touching the toes of other foot) for twelve steps. Repeat two to four times.
- Stand on one foot for thirty seconds. Change foot. Repeat two to four times.

- Standing calf raises: Go from standing flat to on your tiptoes and hold briefly. Repeat eight to twelve times. Rest and repeat.
- Hip extensions: While holding on to the back of a chair, slowly raise your right leg in back of you to about 45 degrees or higher without bending the knee. You can bend your upper body at the waist. Hold briefly and slowly lower your leg. Repeat eight to twelve times with each leg. Rest and repeat.
- Side leg raises: Holding onto a chair, slowly raise your right leg out to the side as far as you can. Keep your knee straight. Hold, then slowly lower your foot to the floor. Do this eight to twelve times. Repeat with your left leg. Rest and repeat with each leg.
- Chair stands: Sit on the front of a sturdy chair with your feet flat on floor. With arms crossed over your chest, hands on your shoulders, stand up slowly and then return to a sitting position slowly. Do eight to twelve repetitions. Rest and repeat.

When each exercise gets too easy, add ankle weights. Start with 1 lb and increase slowly.

RELAXATION EXERCISES

Exercises that relieve tension and promote calm are important for all of us. I have been doing some of these before falling asleep since I learned them in childbirth classes many years ago. There are many ways to clear the clutter from our brain and the tension from our muscles so we can unwind and relax. The following are some suggestions:

- Mindfulness: You can practice this as you do some repetitive tasks such as walking, swimming, or any other active exercise. First focus on your breathing—in through your nose and out through your mouth—and the slow rise and fall of your chest and abdomen. After a few minutes, notice the bigger picture beyond your own body while continuing your slow, rhythmic breathing. Notice the sounds and smells around you. Feel the breeze and note the interplay of light and shadow.

- Meditation can be a source of inner strength and a peaceful way to unwind at the end of a stressful day. Most people need to close their eyes to avoid distraction. Setting aside a special time and place may help. Turn off your phone (land or cell) and get in a relaxed position (e.g., in bed, in a lounger with your feet up and supported). Start with thinking of a peaceful scene (e.g., clouds, the beach, a field, Grandma's house, etc.). Try to recapture the smells you remember or think might be there. Take deep, calming breaths in through the nose and out through pursed lips to slow down your breathing to half the normal rate (eight to ten breaths/minute). Say or think a word or phrase over and over again, like a mantra. Some that come to me include: "I am calm," "I am relaxed," "I am strong," "I can do this," and so on. When you feel distracted, concentrate on your deep breathing until you banish the distractions from your consciousness. This takes practice, but it is worth doing, even for ten minutes. It is a great way to prepare for sleeping.

- Stretching exercises can also be relaxing if you note how your muscle and joints feel as you move them through their range of motion and feel the stretch in the appropriate muscles.

- Progressive muscle relaxation exercises involves alternately tensing and relaxing groups of muscles throughout your body while doing deep breathing in through your nose and out through your mouth. It helps you focus on how each muscle group feels when contracted and when relaxed. These exercises are best done lying down on a mat or a bed in a comfortable position. You can start with the muscles of your face and progress to your feet or start with your feet and ankles and move to your face. I usually start from the top down, but most guided relaxation tapes start from the feet up. As you feel each group of muscles relax, visualize the stress of the day leaving your body while you sink deeper into your mat or mattress. The upper body exercises can be done at your desk multiple times a day to relieve tension.

What Nurses Know...

Each exercise described in this chapter thus far requires practice and repetition to get the maximum benefit. Basic tips for all include starting wherever you find yourself in the physical activity category, from a couch potato to a marathoner. Then slowly take it to the next level. As you become more comfortable with each activity, increase duration, intensity, weights, or other parameters. Start low and increase slowly. If for any reason you have stopped an exercise for longer than a week, resume at a level below where you stopped and progress slowly from there. Overdoing anything may cause pain and injury. Remember, your goal is to develop the lifelong habit of increased physical movement.

BENIFITS OF PHYSICAL ACTIVITY

What do you really get out of increasing your energy output? You might be surprised to learn that you do a lot more than simply burn calories. The following are just some of the benefits of exercise:

- It helps to control weight by increasing muscle tissue and decreasing fat production because the calories eaten are burned more efficiently by your body. When you increase muscle mass (lean tissue) by exercising groups of muscles, you increase your basal metabolic rate (the rate at which you burn calories at rest) even when you are sleeping.
- By exercising heart and lung muscles aerobically, your heart can circulate blood more efficiently, with less effort, and your lungs can take in more oxygen with every breath. The result is that your resting pulse rate and respiratory rate go down and you can relax more completely.

What Nurses Know...

Adequate sun exposure in light-skinned individuals may be as little as ten minutes. Dark-skinned individuals may need sixty minutes or more.

- It increases bone density by providing weight-bearing and muscle tension on long bones (legs and arms). This prevents calcium from leaving bones and improves absorption of calcium. Any outdoor activity increases the manufacture of vitamin D from sun exposure.
- It improves balance and stability because your muscles are increasingly able to correct posture on uneven terrain and keep you from falling. That is more and more important the older one gets.
- It improves digestion and elimination by increasing peristaltic waves and blood flow to the stomach and intestines, thus preventing indigestion and constipation.
- It relaxes blood vessels, thus lowering blood pressure and improving blood flow and oxygenation to all your organs, including your skin (our largest organ) and your brain. So, the more you do, the better you look and the more clearly you can think.
- It increases high-density lipoproteins ("good" cholesterol) and decreases low-density lipoproteins ("bad" cholesterol) and triglycerides, so total cholesterol levels improve. This decreases your risk for heart disease and stroke from the buildup of fatty plaque in arteries.
- It improves sleep patterns by increasing blood flow to muscles, thus removing lactic acid buildup. The more sleep you get, the easier it is to lose weight, the better your immune system is, and the more positive and energetic you are the next day.

Strenuous activity should not be done within three hours of sleep time, because lactic acid may remain in muscle tissue, causing stiffness and pain.

- It enhances your immune system, not only by helping you sleep better and more soundly but also by protecting you from the common cold and from some cancers. Light to moderate consistent exercise causes a temporary boost in the production of macrophages, the cell that gobble up bacteria and viruses. However, too much intense exercise can decrease immunity system function. Stress hormones such as cortisol and adrenaline are produced during extreme exercise, such as running in a marathon or triathlon training. These stress hormones raise blood pressure, blood sugar, and cholesterol levels as well as suppress the immune system.
- It increases a sense of well-being by providing a productive means of getting rid of excess negative emotions, such as anxiety, anger, frustration, and so forth. On the other hand, it increases positive feelings of empowerment and pride in accomplishing a stated goal.
- It even increases libido and performance. Researchers at Harvard Medical School noted in a long-term study that men who exercised thirty minutes a day where forty-one percent less likely to have erectile dysfunction compared with sedentary men. Moderate exercise helps decrease the formation of arterial plaque, thus increasing blood flow to all areas of the body, as noted earlier. For women, the increase in libido is probably due to the increased sense of well-being and positive mood also mentioned earlier.

What Nurses Know...

Physical activity makes muscles more sensitive to insulin, and therefore glucose is used at a much faster rate.

- If all of the benefits just listed are not incentive enough for those of us with diabetes, add the fact that physical activity helps lower blood sugar.

Studies of sedentary individuals have shown that those who engage in regular, low-intensity workouts, such as a ten-minute leisurely stroll, boosted their energy levels by twenty percent and decreased their feelings of fatigue by sixty-five percent compared with individuals who remained sedentary. This is even more important as we age. So, when you come home tired from a too-long and stressful day at work, don't sit in front of the TV to relax and unwind. Change into comfortable clothes and supportive shoes and go for a walk, or actively play with your children or grandchildren, if you have them.

So, what is not to like about increased physical activity?

How Much and How Often?

- The U.S. Department of Health and Human Services 2008 Physical Activity Guidelines for Americans urge most adults to get at least one hundred fifty minutes of moderate aerobic activity or seventy-five minutes of vigorous exercise, or a mixture of each, every week. That works out to twenty to twenty-five minutes of moderate activity or eleven minutes of vigorous exercise, or some combination of the two, per day, divided up in any way that works for you. It's not too difficult if you look at it that way.

What are the differences among light, moderate, and vigorous activity? It depends on how well you can breathe, sweat, and talk while you exercise. Therefore, it is different for everyone and changes as one becomes more fit. During light exercise, you breathe and can talk easily and are not sweating yet. (Of course, in the South, where I live, sweating depends on the weather and whether you are inside or outside.) With moderate exercise you are working harder, breathing faster, and definitely sweating but are still able to talk. (If you are alone, try talking on a cell phone to assess this.) If you indulge in vigorous exercise, you are breathing and sweating hard and find you can talk only in short bursts, if at all. Another way of measuring intensity is to calculate the number of steps per minute. If you are walking slowly, that translates to about eighty steps per minute. Moderate to brisk walking is the equivalent of one hundred steps per minute, whereas fast walking is around one hundred twenty steps per minute, and race walking is more than one hundred twenty steps per minute.

What about pulse rates? There are several ways to look at how fast your pulse rate should be to qualify as aerobic exercise. The easiest method for men is to take your age and subtract it from 220. For women, multiply your age by 0.88 then

What Nurses Know...

As soon as you stop your activity, place your index and middle finger at the side of your neck or over the thumb side of the inside of your wrist and count beats for fifteen seconds. Then multiply by four. An alternative is to count your pulse for ten seconds and multiply by six. This will give you your heart rate per minute after exercising. Do this before you cool down or stretch because, depending on your fitness level, your rate may drop quickly.

subtract that number from 206. The result of either equals your maximum heart rate, which can prove dangerous and should *not* be your goal. Take that number and multiply it by 65% (0.65) and 85% (0.85) to find a safe heart rate range for you. The lower end of the range (65%) is for strengthening the heart, lungs, and circulatory system, and the upper range (85%) is for endurance.

Personally, I try for twenty to thirty minutes of walking per day, more or less, with a heart rate of roughly seventy percent of my maximum, with some strength training and stretching every other day. I am working on adding more balancing exercising to my day to strengthen my core muscles and prevent future falls. It is extremely important that you give yourself permission to not be perfect. We all have good days and some not-so-good days; however, setting realistic goals and scheduling the time are more important than what type of activity we end up doing. As my 91-year-old Swedish friend tells me every time I talk to her, "Every day I wake up in the morning is a good day." Be your own positive influence, or find someone like my friend to inspire you.

How to Increase Your Physical Activity

The following are some tips to help fit more physical activity into your already-busy life:

- Get up a little earlier to go for a walk, run, or bike ride. In fact, why not listen to the morning news while riding a stationary bike?
- Use part of your lunch break to walk or exercise.
- Eat dinner a little earlier to fit in some activity before relaxing for the day.
- Join a gym or a neighborhood sports team. Athletic talent is usually not required.
- Run or walk on an inside or outside track on the way home from work.

- Exercise a dog or actively play with your children or grandchildren, if you have them.
- Vacuum, clean the tile in the bathroom, scrub floors, or perform other household chores. These are very productive activities even if not the most fun things to do. Listening to music or an audio book can make the time fly by.
- Perform any physical activity that you enjoy and is worth your time and energy.
- Make time for you so you can add to or increase your activity level.
- Add ten minutes to a walk around the block, to improve endurance.

Making physical activity a daily routine is as important as going to work or getting to an appointment. Make it a family affair, and get your kids active and away from the TV or the computer. This teaches them that physical activity is important in a well-rounded person. And make it fun. If an incentive to set a specific time for physical activity is needed, remember the old Scottish proverb: "What can be done at *any* time will be done at NO time."

Potential Problems with Exercise

There *is* a downside to physical activity for anyone on insulin or oral medication that makes the pancreas secrete more insulin. That problem is hypoglycemia. Low blood sugar can be avoided, however, by adhering to the following pieces of advice:

1. The best time to be active is about thirty minutes to one hour after a meal. I know what your mother always told you, but unless the activity is prolonged (more than sixty minutes) or very strenuous (swimming fifty laps in an Olympic-size pool), or your meal is loaded with fats and protein (a ten-ounce

What Nurses Know...

When blood sugar is high, it means that the body does not have enough insulin currently in the bloodstream to keep the glucose in the normal range by helping glucose to enter cells. This includes muscle cells, which store glucose as glycogen. When muscle cells are not fed glucose to perform physical activity, they dump stored glycogen into the blood so these muscle cells can burn this glucose. Unfortunately, this use of glucose does not happen because there is insufficient insulin to transport glucose into muscle cells. The end result after exercising with high blood sugar can be an even higher blood glucose level and a very sluggish feeling. When cells cannot get to glucose, fat is burned for energy, resulting in blood and urine ketones.

steak and a large order of fries), you will not get abdominal cramps.

2. When exercise occurs more than two hours after eating, a blood sugar check is in order. If it is less than 120 mg/dl, consider eating or drinking something with about fifteen to thirty milligrams of carbohydrates, such as a piece of fruit, six ounces of orange juice, or an eight-ounce glass of milk. It might be better to take less insulin prior to a meal that precedes planned exercise.

3. Gary Scheiner, author of the book *Think Like a Pancreas*, advised that if your blood sugar is over 250 mg/dl, especially over 350 mg/dl, check your urine for ketones. Ketones are the byproduct of fat metabolism, which indicates that you do not have enough insulin to burn glucose for energy. Postpone exercise until your blood sugar is under 250 mg/dl and ketonuria

is gone. Taking rapid-acting insulin and waiting thirty minutes or so should help.

4. Always carry glucose tablets when taking insulin or oral medication that increases pancreatic secretions. If hypoglycemia unawareness (see Chapter 5) is a problem, exercise with someone who is aware of symptoms and can get help if the need should arise. Carrying a cell phone to call for help is also a good idea.

5. If insulin injections are used, avoid injecting into fatty areas of the extremities used during exercise; for example, if brisk walking, jogging, biking, swimming, or skiing are involved, avoid injecting insulin into the fat over your thigh or buttock muscles. If lifting weights or heavy housecleaning is anticipated, avoid injecting into the back of the upper arms. Exercise increases the blood supply to active muscles, which causes dilatation or widening of smaller blood vessels in the subcutaneous fatty layer directly above these muscles. If insulin has been injected there, it will be absorbed into the bloodstream much faster than usual. This, along with the fact that exercise increases insulin sensitivity of muscles and other tissue, makes hypoglycemia even more likely.

6. Check your blood sugar a couple of hours after physical activity, because an intense workout may cause hypoglycemia for several hours. Making the body more insulin sensitive has its drawbacks if the usual amount of insulin or oral medication is taken and exercise is added. It may be wise to discuss with your healthcare practitioner reducing medication on days when planned exercise is prolonged and/or strenuous, or eating more carbs in order to prevent a low blood sugar. (See John's comment at the beginning of this chapter.)

7. Before starting an exercise program, check with your healthcare professional, who may order an exercise stress test to see how your heart and blood pressure respond. If diabetic

complications are in the picture, see common restrictions and alternative suggestions listed here:

Complications*	Exercise to Avoid	Rationale	Choose Instead
Peripheral neuropathy	Jogging Brisk walking Climbing	May cause foot trauma, turned ankles, falls	Swimming Stationary bike Rowing machine
Autonomic neuropathy	Strenuous or prolonged exercise	Decreased cardiovascular response, postural hypotension	Walking Swimming Treadmill
Proliferative retinopathy	Jogging Skiing Body contact sports Any jarring or rapid head movement Heavy lifting Any use of breath-holding	May cause retinal detachment or hemorrhage in the back of the eye	Walking Swimming Stationary bike
Nephropathy	Strenuous or prolonged exercise	May increase proteinuria. Does not affect progression of renal disease	Walking Swimming Exercise equipment for mild to moderate intensity and duration
Cardiovascular disease, including congestive heart failure & hypertension	Heavy lifting, any use of breath-holding, strenuous or prolonged exercise	May cause angina, arrhythmias, & increased blood pressure if not well controlled	Swimming Treadmill Stationary bike

With permission from Mertig, RG, *The Nurse's Guide to Teaching Diabetes Self-Management*, Springer Publishing Company, LLC, New York, NY.
*See Chapter 6 for further discussion of complications.

What Nurses Know...

Peripheral neuropathy is a condition whereby nerve supply to an area, such as the toes, skin of feet, or sole or heel of the foot is diminished or nonexistent and so any irritation (e.g., the friction from a stone, or a nail, etc.) is not felt. In addition, adequate blood supply is needed to heal and prevent infection even with a minor wound. Any injured skin and tissue should be reported to a healthcare practitioner immediately.

8. Adequate hydration is important for everyone, whether you exercise or not. However, it is even more important for all individuals to drink water before and after exercising. If physical activity is very strenuous or prolonged, fluid intake *during* exercise is also important to prevent dehydration from excessive perspiration. Water is the best choice for fluid replacement. Sports drinks contain calories, sugar, and electrolytes, which are usually needed only by endurance athletes.

9. Inspect your feet after exercise to check for blisters and/or reddened areas. This is especially important for individuals with decreased nerve sensations and/or blood supply to the feet, who may not feel the injury.

10. It goes without saying that good supportive shoes, moisture-wicking socks, and comfortable clothing are a must. Checking the inside of shoes for worn areas or small items that may cause discomfort or injury is important for everyone. My nondiabetic husband once realized his foot was sharing a shoe with an insect and now always looks before slipping his feet into shoes.

Those of us with diabetes need to be reminded that healthy lifestyle choices are a must for everyone and not an imposition as a result of having diabetes. Increasing physical activity is important for everyone of any age. All adults should *try* to achieve the recommended 10,000 steps a day. This is a goal, not an absolute. Inexpensive pedometers and aerobic monitors are easily found in drug and variety stores. Recording your activity level is both empowering and motivating. Some monitors equate steps taken with calories burned and miles walked. Because every step counts, a step counter may provide the encouragement to take the stairs instead of the elevator or to walk to do errands, especially if today is turning out to be a low-step day. Given the examples above of how physical activity impacts our lives in so many positive ways, we need to *just do it!*

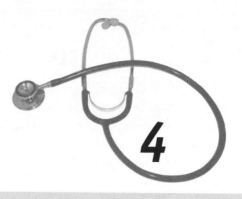

4

How Do Medications Help?

I told my doctor that ever since he said I had type 2 diabetes I have tried my best to lose weight and walk two to three times a week, but my morning blood sugar is always 200 or more. I feel tired all the time, and I am very discouraged. I want to feel good again. What else can I do?   JUDY

When lifestyle changes such as healthy eating, weight loss, and exercise are not enough to normalize blood sugars, there is always medication to consider as an option. Just like Judy, many people with diabetes are frustrated and discouraged. You want your old, life (before diabetes) back. Most of you with type 2 diabetes don't realize that you may not have felt really good for awhile before the diagnosis of diabetes. Yes, you are getting older, but diabetes didn't just happen. You probably had prediabetes for a few years as your blood glucose levels were rising higher and higher. Maybe you got sleepy after a high-carb meal but thought, don't most people need a nap after dinner? So here you are a few months after diagnosis, and now you are ready to do more to control those darn blood sugars. Lucky for you there are many choices of medication today. If one doesn't work, there are others, and most can be combined, if needed, to improve effectiveness. So, what do you need to know about possible medications and their side effects? Well, this chapter is a primer on the various types. If this list seems overwhelming, just look at the drug that your healthcare practitioner has prescribed and save the rest for later.

The classifications of oral drugs and types of insulin have expanded exponentially in the last fifteen years. Diabetes is big business, and pharmaceutical companies are leading the pack to cash in. Besides new medications, we now have combinations of medications that complement each other in one pill. So much has happened so quickly that it is confusing and difficult for healthcare professionals and the public to keep up. Newer, more powerful, and useful drugs come on the market with dizzying frequency. The companies that make these drugs, and the Web addresses of each, are listed in the Resources section at the end of this book so you can do further research. It will be several years before the patents of the newer drugs expire and their generic equivalents become available. That means that the latest and often best medications are very expensive. Many of the pharmaceutical companies have programs for providing their new drugs for free or at reduced cost to people who meet certain criteria, so if you are having difficulty buying your necessary medications, go to one of the following Web sites:

1. Partnership for Prescription Assistance: www.pparx.org 1-888-4PPA-NOW (477-2669)
2. National Diabetes Information Clearing House: http://diabetes.niddk.nih.gov/dm/pubs/financialhelp
3. Free Medicines: http://freemedicine.com/index.htm1-573-996-3333

4. Access to Wellness: www.access2wellness.com/a2w/index.
   html1-866-317-2775
5. Astra Zeneca: www.rxassist.org/
6. SelectCare Benefits Network: www.scbn.org/index.html1-888-
   331-1002

To receive assistance from one of these groups you must be referred through your healthcare provider. Asking your provider about this service may start the ball rolling. In addition, an Internet search of any drug trade name or generic will result in a list of Web sites with information for you and your healthcare professional. For older drugs, try searching www.webmd.com.

Oral Antidiabetic Medications

Oral medications that help to lower blood glucose levels do so in a number of different ways. They may stimulate your pancreas to increase its production of insulin; decrease insulin resistance in cells and tissue so your own insulin production works better; or slow intestinal absorption of carbohydrates so the rise in blood glucose takes place over a longer period of time, giving your own insulin time to move it out of the bloodstream. There are also many combinations of different drugs to accomplish more than one of these actions.

MEDS THAT INCREASE INSULIN PRODUCTION

Secretagogues are drugs that make the pancreas increase its production of insulin. Four classes of secretagogues are currently in use: (1) sulfonylureas, (2) meglitinides, (3) D-phenylalanine derivatives, and (4) dipeptidyl peptidase-4 (DPP-4) inhibitors. They are prescribed only for persons with type 2 diabetes because type 1 diabetics do not produce insulin any more. Because they all work a little differently, I discuss them separately.

Sulfonylureas   Sulfonylureas were the first and only oral antidiabetic drugs for type 2 diabetics for many years. The only first-generation sulfonylurea still on the market is Diabinese, which is rarely used today. Second- and third-generation drugs are more potent and so can be given at lower dosages. They also have fewer side effects than the first-generation drugs, although low blood sugar is still a possibility when meals are not eaten or delayed or exercise is prolonged. They may also cause weight gain, water retention, and sometimes flushing if alcoholic beverages are drunk, although this is less common than with Diabinese. The weight gain is an especially vexing problem, because increased weight increases insulin resistance. Water retention can also increase blood pressure, which is often a part of the diabetic picture. Sulfonylureas should be prescribed only for type 2 clients who are able to increase their beta cell production of insulin. Because type 2 diabetes is a progressive disease, eventually the beta cells will have no more to give, and different drugs, including insulin, may be added or substituted to bring blood glucose into a normal range. Sulfonylureas are also mild sulfa drugs that may not be appropriate for individuals who may be allergic to such drugs. The following is a list of newer sulfonylureas along with their generic name. Drug names marked with an asterisk are currently available in generic form (generic names are in parentheses), with more to be added as patents expire.

Glucotrol* (glipizide) and Glucatrol XL* (glipizide ER)
DiaBeta* (glyburide)
Glynase PresTab* (micronized glyburide)
Micronase (glyburide)
Amaryl* (glimepiride)

Meglitinides The only drug approved by the Food and Drug Administration (FDA) to date in this class is repaglinide (Prandin). Its mechanism of action is similar to sulfonylureas; however, it acts much more rapidly. Therefore, it should be taken right before a meal. It increases insulin production dependent on carbohydrates from this meal. This increases the flexibility of meal planning and decreases incidence of low blood sugar because it should not be taken if you are not planning to each within thirty minutes. It can be taken alone or combined with metformin, alpha-glucosidase inhibitors, or thiazolidinediones (TZDs).

D-Phenylalanine Derivatives The only FDA-approved drug in this class is nateglinide (Starlix), which acts similarly to Prandin in that it stimulates a rapid release of insulin from the beta cells, thus controlling blood sugars after meals. It also should be taken right before a meal, so the side effect of low blood sugar is rare. Because it is broken down and partially excreted by the liver, its duration of action can be prolonged if you have significant liver disease, resulting in an increased risk of hypoglycemia. This drug can be taken alone or in combination with metformin to make the body tissues more insulin sensitive.

Dipeptidyl Peptidase-4 Inhibitors This is the newest class of drugs that increase the amount of insulin produced by the pancreas, but this increase occurs after meals, when blood glucose tends to be high. They are taken once a day, with or without food, at the same time of day. These drugs can be taken alone or in combination with metformin. They should not be taken with another secretagogue such as those listed earlier. Side effects include low blood sugar if meals are skipped. These drugs may also cause a stuffy or runny nose; sore throat; headache; painful, burning urination; stomach pain; nausea; vomiting; diarrhea; and bloating. Examples of DPP-4 inhibitors include: (1) Januvia (sitagliptin), (2) Onglyza (saxagliptin), and (3) Janumet (sitagliptin and metformin).

MEDICATIONS THAT DECREASE INSULIN RESISTANCE
Biguanides Drugs in this class act primarily to decrease the liver's inappropriate release of glycogen into the blood, thus increasing blood sugar. It also improves tissue insulin sensitivity, both problems in type 2 diabetes. Metformin (Glucophage) was the first nonsulfonylurea to be added to the arsenal of oral

What Nurses Know...

Lactic acidosis is a form of acidosis (too much acid in the blood) caused by decreased oxygenation of cells. Lactate is cleared from blood, primarily by the liver, with the kidneys (10-20%) and skeletal muscles to a lesser degree. All metformin formulations, including the newer ones and combinations with metformin in them, have a black box warning for this reason. If you have a problem with liver or kidney disease, you should not take this drug.

drugs for type 2 diabetes. Side effects, which decrease over time, include diarrhea, bloating, and nausea. They can be minimized by taking the lowest dose and increasing it slowly if needed until you have good glycemic control. The most problematic side effect is lactic acidosis, which is rare but can be fatal.

All metformin formulations, including the newer ones and combinations with metformin in them, have a black box warning for this reason. If you have a problem with liver or kidney disease, you should not take this drug. When taken alone, Glucophage does not contribute to weight gain or cause low blood sugar. It may even lower low-density lipoprotein ("bad" cholesterol) and triglyceride levels, which can be problems with type 2 diabetes. This drug can be used as a first-line medication to improve glucose control, or it can be combined with a sulfonylurea, meglitinides (e.g., Prandin), alpha-glucosidase inhibitors (Precose and Glyset), a TZD (Actos and Avandia), or insulin.

Six combination pills are currently available: (1) Glucovance (metformin and glyburide; currently available in generic form), (2) Metaglip (metformin and glipizide; currently available in generic form), (3) Avandamet (metformin and Avandia), (4)

What Nurses Know...

First-line drugs are those that can be prescribed first as a drug of choice when medication needs to be added to diet and exercise to normalize blood glucose levels.

Actoplus Met (metformin and Actos), (5) Janumet (metformin and Januvia), and (6) PrandiMet (metformin and Prandin). As the rate of type 2 diabetes increases, more drug companies will add to the available combinations. Combination drugs increase ease of use and compliance as well as cost. The two separate medications may currently both be available as generics, but the newer combination may not be available as a generic for several years.

Newer drugs in the same class as Glucophage include Glumetza and Fortamet, which are extended-release formulations of metformin for the treatment of type 2 diabetes. They are actually metformin derivatives that may have fewer side effects

What Nurses Know...

Metformin alone or in any of its combinations can interfere with the absorption of vitamin B-12, which is needed for red cell production and to keep nerve cells healthy. Continue to get lab work done yearly, which should help identify anemia, and tell your healthcare provider if you begin to lose sensation in your feet.

than metformin and are taken only once a day. Riomet is a liquid formulation of metformin for children and those who have difficulty swallowing pills.

The following is a list of drugs currently available in the biguanides class. Those marked with an asterisk are available in generic form. Generic names are in parentheses.

Glucophage* (metformin) and Glucophage XR (metformin ER)
Glumetza (metformin extended release)
Fortamet (metformin extended release)
Riomet (metformin oral solution)
Glucovance* (metformin and glyburide)
Metaglip* (metformin and glipizide)
Avandamet (metformin and rosiglitazone)
Actoplus Met (metformin and pioglitazone)
Janumet (metformin and sitagliptin)
PrandiMet (metformin and repaglinide)

Thiazolidinediones This group of drugs, better known as *glitazones*, or TZDs, includes pioglitazone (Actos) and rosiglitazone (Avandia). They act by decreasing the tissues' resistance to insulin, thus improving control of blood sugars. These can be taken in conjunction with sulfonylureas, meglitinides (Prandin), metformin (Glucophage or Avandamet), alpha-glucosidase inhibitors (Precose or Glyset), or insulin. The FDA recommends that liver function tests be done before and during treatment with this class of drugs because the first TZD, troglitazon (Rezulin), was withdrawn from the market in 2000 because of reports of rare incidents of liver failure and related deaths. The two newer drugs, Actos and Avandia, are much less toxic to the liver. If you are taking a TZD and your liver enzymes increase, you are usually taken off this class of drugs and put on some other medication.

Glitazone drugs can also cause fluid retention and rapid weight gain independent of fluid retention. If you are at risk for congestive heart failure, you should probably not take this class of drugs. Everyone taking these medications needs to be monitored for heart function and weight gain, ruling out fluid retention as the cause. Medications in this class, including combinations drugs, have a black box warning concerning heart failure and heart muscle ischemia (inadequate blood supply).

If you are also taking drugs to lower cholesterol, the name of the anticholesterol medication should be listed in your medical chart so that certain drug interactions do not occur. For example, cholestyramine (Questran) inhibits the absorption of TZDs as well as other drugs and should not be taken at the same time. Also, it may take several weeks or months to see the full effect of Actos or Avandia, so you should monitor blood glucose levels at least once a day or more often and keep a record to show your healthcare practitioner. If you are taking insulin or a secret-

What Nurses Know...

In June 2010, two teams of researchers, after conducting studies with large numbers of patients, concluded that Avandia increases the risk of heart disease, heart failure, stroke, and death in people who take this drug to help control diabetes. On September 23, 2010, the FDA put severe restrictions on the use of Avandia. Any healthcare professional prescribing this drug must state that everything else has failed to control blood sugars and that clients understand the substantial risks to the heart this drug poses. If you take Avandia alone or in a combination drug, your healthcare provider will probably switch you to another diabetes drug soon. Actos, the only other TZD on the market, affects a different set of genes and is considered safe.

agogue during this time, the dose may need to be lowered as the TZD kicks in.

Two new combination drugs, Avandaryl and Duetact, are now on the market. These drugs combine Avandia or Actos with glimepiride, a third-generation sulfonylurea (brand name Amaryl). It has the same precautions concerning liver function and should be administered with the first good meal of the day to minimize low blood sugar from Amaryl.

MEDICINES THAT SLOW INTESTINAL ABSORPTION OF CARBOHYDRATES

Alpha-Glucosidase Inhibitors   The two drugs in this class, acarbose (Precose; called Glucobay in Europe and Prandase in Canada) and miglitol (Glyset), work in the small intestine to delay and/ or block the digestion of carbohydrates (starches and sucrose) and decrease the peak postprandial (after meals) glucose levels, allowing insulin production to better match glucose absorption. They can be taken alone or in combination with sulfonylureas, repaglinide (Prandin), metformin (Glucophage), TZDs (Actos or Avandia), or insulin. When taken alone, these drugs do not cause hypoglycemia, but when taken with other agents that do cause

What Nurses Know . . .

If you take Precose or Glyset AND a drug that increases insulin production, you may develop low blood sugar. If you do, your usual ways of treating this will not work; for example, table sugar, honey, LifeSavers, milk, and anything sweetened with these ingredients will not be absorbed to raise glucose levels. You must take something with glucose, such as glucose tablets or a gel pack.

low blood sugar only glucose (in the form of glucose tablets or gel) or fructose from fruit juice will treat the low blood sugar.

The most common side effects of Precose and Glyset are gas, diarrhea, and cramps. These get better with time and are minimized by starting at the lowest dose and gradually increasing it if needed to control blood sugars. Because of these side effects, this drug may not be appropriate for you if you also have irritable bowel syndrome.

Injectable Antidiabetic Medication

As long as I could take a pill, I could accept the diagnosis of diabetes. After all, it was just like taking my vitamin pill. No big deal, right? But when the doctor said I had to take insulin, I really freaked out. No needles, please! I'll do anything to avoid sticking myself. Too late. Insulin it is. KEVIN

You may have reacted to the need to take insulin just as Kevin did. When you look at the side effects of some of the drugs listed earlier, however, you may decide that taking insulin, a hormone made by the body, may be a better deal after all. The bottom line in your thinking should be: Do whatever it takes to keep blood glucose levels as close to normal as possible, even if that means taking insulin. The good news is if you have type 2 diabetes, weight loss of even ten to twenty pounds may mean that you can come

What Nurses Know . . .

Hypoglycemia is the same as low blood sugar.
Hyperglycemia is the same as high blood sugar.

off of insulin and maybe need only diet and exercise to keep your blood sugars straight. So take heart and read on.

INSULIN

The body needs insulin 24/7. When the islet cells of the pancreas perform as intended, a small amount of endogenous (originating from within the body) insulin is secreted constantly to allow some glucose to enter cells for cellular function. When we inject exogenous (originating outside the body) insulin for this purpose, we refer to it as a *basal insulin.* As the normal islet cells sense a rise in blood sugar from a meal or snack, the beta cells produce more endogenous insulin to keep blood sugar within the normal range. We can give bolus doses of exogenous insulin prior to eating to mimic this activity when the pancreas is not able to do so. The two purposes of insulin therapy are (1) to maximize glycemic control while minimizing the risk of hypoglycemia and (2) to effectively mimic the body's physiologic need for insulin as both a basal and a bolus amount.

Tight glucose control, especially using insulin, has been shown in several clinical trials to prevent or delay the onset of complications caused by high blood sugars. The unintended consequence of keeping blood sugars at near-normal levels is low blood sugar. The pancreas, when it is healthy, does a much better job at doing this than the human brain, even aided by a glucose meter and multiple insulin injections or the use of an insulin pump. However, with effort and the right combination of

What Nurses Know...

A1c is a blood test that measures the average percentage of blood glucose over a two- to three-month period.

insulins, clients with type 1 and type 2 diabetes can achieve close to normal glycemic control as measured by hemoglobin A1c with minimal hypoglycemic episodes.

Obviously, all of us with type 1 diabetes take a basal insulin that keeps our body functioning between meals and throughout the night and a bolus insulin dose before meals. Basal insulins can consist of

1. one dose per day of a long-acting insulin,
2. two doses of an intermediate-acting insulin, or
3. various basal rates with rapid-acting insulin using an insulin pump.

Bolus doses of insulin, on the other hand, cover episodes of hyperglycemia and meal or snack carbohydrate amounts and are given as needed. This is much easier to do with an insulin pump, but it also can be managed by giving injections of rapid-acting insulin prior to a meal or snack. Additional insulin can be added or subtracted on the basis of the current blood sugar level. For instance, a person might start with a sliding scale for rapid-acting insulin to take care of higher than normal blood sugar prior to meals. A set ratio of units of insulin to grams of carbohydrates (see the "Carbohydrate Counting" section in Chapter 2) would be added to the sliding scale amount to minimize the effect of the meal or snack on blood sugar. Examples of insulin to carbohydrate ratios might resemble one of the following:

One unit of insulin for every ten grams of carbohydrate
One unit of insulin for every twelve grams of carbohydrate
One unit of insulin for every fifteen grams of carbohydrate
One unit of insulin for every twenty grams of carbohydrate

This ratio may be different at each meal or may remain the same. If this sounds difficult, it can be. The troubling aspect of working all of this out is that each one of us responds to food and insulin differently, so it is a matter of trial and error. Because each person is different, you have to be self-reliant and willing to experiment. Only those of us committed to our long-term survival with the desire to live as normal a life as possible will be able to handle this challenge. It also helps to have a diabetes educator on your team who is willing to troubleshoot any problems and answer your many questions. See Chapter 9 for more about getting the help you need.

Insulin therapy for those of you with type 2 diabetes is gaining more interest. Because hyperglycemia has such devastating consequences over time, glycemic control needs to be achieved as soon as possible. Insulin should not be used as a last resort in treating type 2 diabetes or as an indication that all attempts with oral drugs have failed. It should never be used as a threat or punishment for those of you who may be labeled *noncompliant* with weight loss and lifestyle changes. It may be the treatment of choice for some of you with type 2 diabetes right from the start. According to the American Diabetes Association, insulin should be used in treating type 2 diabetes when

1. Hyperglycemia is severe at diagnosis
2. Glycemic control is not achieved with lifestyle changes and combinations of oral meds

What Nurses Know...

The burning of fat for energy when there is not enough insulin to push glucose into cells causes ketones to build up in the blood (ketonemia) and the kidneys excrete them in the urine (ketonuria).

3. Uncontrolled hyperglycemia is caused by infection, acute injury, surgery, heart attack, stroke, or other cardiovascular incident
4. The above incidents cause ketonemia and/or ketonuria and uncontrolled weight loss
5. Liver and/or renal disease complicate metabolism and excretion of oral antidiabetic medications
6. Pregnancy is a contraindication to the use of some oral anti-diabetic drugs

The American Diabetes Association also recommends that the use of insulin be viewed in the same light as all noninsulin drugs for individuals with type 2 diabetes and that more people be started on insulin alone or in combination with metformin or other nonsecretagogues sooner rather than later. If glycemic control is delayed, the risk of developing chronic complications (see Chapter 6) is increased. The sooner blood sugars are controlled, the better.

Types of Insulin   Insulin was discovered in the 1920s and at that time consisted of a short-acting insulin distillate from the pancreas of dogs. Children with type 1 diabetes needed injections every four to five hours, even during the night. In the 1940s, protamine was added to regular insulin to make NPH (proto-mine hagedorn) insulin, and zinc was added to regular insulin to make lente insulin. This slowed the onset, peak, and, most important, duration of insulin and decreased the number of injections needed per day.

Prior to 1985, insulin came from the pancreases of cows and pigs and was marketed as beef, beef-pork, or purified porcine insulin. Porcine insulin was the closest in molecular structure to endogenous human insulin. The use of insulin from different species gave rise to allergic reactions, immunologic suppression of this insulin's action, and the fear that there would not be sufficient animal pancreases to meet the increasing need for insulin therapy. Most insulin used today in the United States is called *human insulin* and is manufactured in a laboratory using recombinant DNA technology. If enough regular insulin is given to keep two-hour postprandial blood sugar under 140 mg/dl, this often causes a low blood sugar three to four hours later. The minimum thirty-minute delay in eating after the insulin dose is often a problem as well. Regular insulin, although the shortest acting insulin we had for decades, just does not match the increase in blood sugar generated by a typical meal. Its duration of action is also too long, causing frequent between-meal hypoglycemic reactions. To mimic the around-the-clock action of the body's insulin, intermediate and long-acting insulins were developed as previously described. Until 2005, NPH, lente, and ultralente insulins were available from both major companies that manufacture insulin in the United States: Eli Lilly and

What Nurses Know...

The following steps outline proper disposal of insulin syringes, pen needles, lancets, and pump insertion needles (anything sharp):

1. Get a red biohazard container for this purpose from the health department if required by state or district laws.
2. Use an opaque, nonpiercable container with a narrow opening, such as a bleach bottle. When three quarters full, seal the cap on with glue or layers of duct tape.
3. Never throw used needles, even with caps on, into the trash for IV drug users to find or trash handlers to stick themselves with, causing fear of HIV or other infectious diseases.

Novo Nordisk. Both have stopped making lente and ultralente because the rapid and long-acting insulin analogs have supplanted their use. Each company also makes combination vials of NPH and regular human insulins for use in syringes and with their cartridge-filled pens.

Insulin Analogs   The new rapid-acting insulin analogs have had a huge impact on controlling postprandial hyperglycemia and/or hypoglycemia. Insulin analogs are not human insulin; they are better. By rearranging some amino acids on human insulin's protein molecular structure, a faster onset and peak and shortened duration have been achieved. The result is an insulin that more closely matches the rise of blood sugar caused by a meal or snack. There are three rapid-acting insulin analogs in current use—insulin lispro (Humalog), insulin aspart (Novolog), and insulin glulisine (Apidra)—all of which are used for bolus dosing and can be used in insulin pumps or combined in a syringe with intermediate-acting insulin analogs for basal coverage. All rapid-acting insulin analogs can be used by type 1 and type 2 diabetics and injected or administered via insulin pump. All insulin analogs require a prescription and client education regarding their use, especially if the you have any experience with short-acting regular insulin. Regular and NPH insulins as well as their various combinations do not require a prescription, although for health insurance coverage one may be needed. Some states require that a person sign for insulin sold without a prescription, to provide a record.

If rearranging amino acids can accelerate the action of human insulin, why can't different arrangements prolong the action? The first truly long-acting basal insulin was made by doing just that a few years ago. We now have two such basal insulin analogs, insulin glargine (Lantus), and, the latest, insulin detemir (Levemir). These analogs are described as "peakless" and may be used with rapid or short-acting insulin in treating type 1 and type 2 diabetes. They may also be used as a basal insulin with secretagogues or other oral agents for type 2 glycemic control. Both Lantus and Levemir require a prescription. If you are using either of these two long-acting analogs, DO NOT mix them with other insulins in the same syringe. You must be willing to give two separate injections when using a basal insulin analog in conjunction with rapid or short-acting insulin. Both types of insulin may, however, be given at the same time, but in separate syringes. Both insulin glargine and insulin detemir improve fasting blood sugars and reduce the variability of peak action association with ultralente and NPH intermediate-acting insulins. They can both be administered to children as young as six years old with type 1 diabetes.

Eli Lilly makes a premixed insulin, Humalog Mix 75/25, with 75% lispro protamine suspension and 25% insulin lispro and a humulog mix 50/50. Novo Nordisk's premixed insulin, NovoLog 70/30, contains 70% aspart protamine and 30% insulin aspart. All analog mixtures require a prescription and are available in vials for syringe use and cartridges for each company's insulin pens, manufactured for your convenience.

How to Measure and Inject Insulin   Insulin syringes come in several sizes, from 1 cc with a 100-unit capacity; a low-dose syringe, with a 50-unit capacity, and the smallest, with a 30-unit capacity. Use the smallest syringe that will accommodate the amount of insulin you are taking. In order to draw up liquid from a vial you must first inject the same amount of air into the vial to overcome the vacuum. If you are mixing regular (clear) insulin and NPH (cloudy) insulin in the same syringe, you must avoid getting any cloudy solution into the clear. Follow these rules:

1. Draw up air into the syringe to match the amount of regular insulin and inject it into the vial of regular insulin and remove the syringe.
2. Draw up air into the same syringe to match the amount of NPH insulin and inject into the vial of NPH insulin then remove syringe.
3. Draw up the correct amount of regular insulin (clear).

What Nurses Know . . .

Avoid injecting into the area that you will exercise soon after-ward. For example, do not inject into the fat over your thighs if you plan to walk or run afterward. This will increase the blood supply to thigh muscles and increase the absorption rate for the fatty tissue above and could cause low blood sugar.

4. Add the correct amount of NPH insulin (cloudy) to the regular insulin in the syringe. The total amount should equal the amount of regular insulin plus the amount of NPH insulin.

Give injections in the fatty areas of the abdomen, avoiding a one-inch area around the navel, the back of the upper arm (use a door jamb to roll the fat forward so you can see it), the front of the thigh, and the upper part of the buttocks. Leave about a one-inch space between injection sites, and rotate between areas with each injection. If you administer more than one injection a day, make a plan to rotate between sites that is based on how much time you have between an injection and eating. Insulin injected into the abdomen is absorbed the fastest, and next fastest from the arms. The thighs have a slower absorption rate, and the slowest absorption is from the buttocks. One day use the right side, and the next day the left. Giving injections in the same area over and over again will create scar tissue and decrease the absorption rate after awhile.

Pinch up the fat and angle the needle from thirty to ninety degrees, depending on the depth of the fat. For more information about insulin injection sites, go to www.lillydiabetes.com/content/insulin-injections.jsp.

Insulin Pumps   Until there is either a cure for diabetes or an affordable, reliable, internal artificial pancreas, an insulin pump is the next best thing. Characteristics of a person who would do well pumping insulin include someone

1. On intensive insulin therapy (three or more injections per day) but not meeting glycemic goals
2. Able and willing to make appropriate insulin adjustments based on frequent blood sugar testing
3. Well motivated to learn pump technology and able to follow through and make the necessary changes
4. Wanting or requiring a more flexible lifestyle with regard to meals and exercise
5. Willing to be tethered via tubing to a small box housing a continuous flow of rapid-acting insulin (except for the OmniPod, which is wireless and disposable)
6. With added incentive to control blood sugar prior to and during pregnancy,
7. With adequate health insurance to help with cost
8. Perhaps most important, with a take-charge personality who is willing to do whatever it takes to make it work

Pumping insulin is definitely worth the hassles involved. When I was put on my first insulin pump after working at blood sugar control for ten years with four to five injections a day, I felt like I finally had my life back. I could eat and exercise when I wanted without worrying about when my intermediate-acting insulin was going to peak. When the insulin analogs became available, insulin decision making became even easier. I could eat what I wanted, when I wanted, within reason, just like anyone else. However, monitoring blood glucose levels to set basal rates throughout the day and night meant pre- and postprandial testing as well as testing two or three times during the night. Pumping insulin is not the answer for everyone. It takes effort, a willingness to experiment, and the ability to follow through in order to use an insulin pump successfully. Blood sugars usually level out so that the roller coaster ride of highs and lows, often in the same day, rarely occurs. Blood sugars are more predictable and food, physical activity, and insulin doses finally make sense.

Deciding to go on an insulin pump does have its aggravations. Pump alarms for low volume, low battery, and "no delivery" are important safety precautions but can be embarrassing. However, they can usually be set to vibrate. The "no delivery" alarm must be tended to very quickly because very high blood sugars and diabetic ketoacidosis can ensue in a matter of a few hours. Most pumpers use rapid-acting insulin analogs in their pumps, which have a very short duration of action. Tubing, reservoirs, and insulin must be readily available at work and at home, as well as anywhere that you might be, for this potential emergency. A low battery is less problematic, because most pumps will continue to function for eight or more hours. A pump rarely malfunctions, but the 1-800 number on the back of the pump is manned 24/7 to help you troubleshoot problems and reprogram the pump, if needed. It is probably wise to keep an up-to-date written record of all basal rates so they can be reset. If there is a delay in fixing any glitch, syringes and insulin must be available as backup.

That brings us to the "stuff" that pump users need to carry with them. Anyone diagnosed with type 1 or type 2 diabetes should carry medication that must be taken with meals as well as a glucose monitor, strips, a lancing device and lancets, tissues, a log book, and spare batteries for the monitor. Most monitors come with convenient carrying cases for that purpose. In addition, anyone on insulin should have available unexpired insulin, syringes, and alcohol swabs. Pumpers also need extra reservoirs and tubing, fresh pump batteries, and any other paraphernalia needed to change the insulin setup and/or insertion site. There are coolers, pouches, and carrying cases for this purpose. Supplies can also be carried in a purse, backpack, fanny pack, or briefcase. If not refrigerated, insulin at room temperature will maintain its potency for at least twenty-eight days. Do not, however, freeze or leave insulin in 90-degree weather. Leaving insulin in the glove compartment of a car, even in spring or fall, is a bad idea.

Most people who use insulin pumps use the abdomen as their insertion site, upper abdomen for men and lower abdomen for women. However, all appropriate subcutaneous sites for insulin injection, such as the front of the thigh, back of the upper arm, and upper buttocks, can be used. The insertion site should be changed every two to three days to prevent irritation and infection. Pumps can be disconnected for bathing, swimming, contact sports, and sexual activity for up to two hours if blood sugars are well controlled. When reconnected, you should monitor your blood sugar, and an appropriate bolus dose, if needed, should be given.

Persons using insulin pumps need a support system, both professionally and personally. A supportive diabetes educator and/or endocrinologist can help troubleshoot any pump and/ or blood sugar difficulties. Selected family members, friends, and/or coworkers should be informed as to how they can help in meaningful ways. This may mean that they demonstrate their concern by asking about blood sugars/meal preferences, providing privacy and a regular Coke or other fast-acting sugar source when hypoglycemia is a problem, or none of the above except when asked. Wearing an insulin pump is a serious financial and personal commitment to controlling blood sugars and managing diabetes while decreasing hypoglycemic episodes and increasing lifestyle flexibility. Insulin pumps are appropriate not only for type 1 diabetes but also for type 2. Children as young as age one year can also be managed well with an insulin pump. Parents can set lock-out controls so that young children cannot change settings.

OTHER INJECTABLE DIABETES MEDICATION

Two new types of subcutaneous (in the fatty tissue under the skin) injectable medications have been recently added to the arsenal of drugs to control blood sugar: (1) pramlintide (Symlin) and (2) a group of drugs classified as *incretin mimetics.*

Amylin Hormone   Pramlintide is a synthetic amylin hormone that is normally produced by the beta cells of the pancreas, as is insulin. Pramlintide injections given with meals that contain at least two hundred fifty calories and thirty grams of carbohydrates should not cause hypoglycemia or weight gain, as insulin does, and may even promote weight loss. It should be given with rapid-acting insulin at meals but cannot be mixed in the same syringe. The amount of rapid-acting insulin given before a meal may even be lowered by fifty percent. Symlin also comes in 60-mcg (for type 1 diabetics) and 120-mcg (for type 2 diabetics) prefilled pens. After the beginning of 2011, Symlin will be available only as SymlinPen. This will be more convenient, eliminate confusion regarding dosing, and prevent the possibility of mixing it with insulin. Because Symlin is dosed in micrograms, it should never be withdrawn from the pen into a syringe. This could result in a higher dose. Pens should be refrigerated but never frozen. The pen in current use should be kept cool (under 77°F). Discard an opened pen after 30 days even if it still contains medication. The SymlinPen comes in packages of two per box, requires a prescription, and is light sensitive, so keep it in the box in which it came. Like all pen delivery systems, needles are sold separately and are screwed onto the pen at the time of delivery. Very short needles are available for injection in the fatty layer under the skin just as insulin is. After injecting the medication, remove the needle and return the pen to the box and place into the refrigerator or cooler. The benefits of Symlin include the following:

- It decreases after meal elevations of blood glucose. If you are using this drug, you should test your blood sugar before meals, two hours after meals, and at bedtime.
- It smooths out blood sugar levels throughout the day, with fewer blood sugar swings.
- It improves your A1c test results.
- It helps you need less insulin.

• It helps you feel full sooner at meals, so you may eat less. This may help you lose weight.

Obviously, this drug is not for everyone. Symlin has been approved for use for people with both type 1 and type 2 diabetes using rapid-onset insulin as a premeal bolus dose who are not achieving glycemic control on their present regimen and are well motivated to follow directions carefully. The most common side effect is nausea, which improves after a few weeks. The dose is started low and is gradually increased until the desired effect is achieved.

Incretin Mimetic   The second new class of injectable medications for treating type 2 diabetes is called an *incretin mimetic*. This is a synthetic version of the human incretin hormone GLP-1 (glucagon-like peptide-1) that is secreted in the small intestines, but it lasts longer. The first drug in this class is Byetta (exenatide), which helps the body to self-regulate glycemic control. It enhances insulin secretion only when blood sugar is elevated and decreases insulin production as blood sugar normalizes. According to its manufacturer, this drug is for persons with type 2 diabetes who are taking metformin or a sulfonylurea or both without achieving glycemic control. Byetta is used in conjunction with these medications, although the dose of metformin and/or sulfonylurea may need to be reduced. Byetta is dispensed in prefilled thirty-day supply pens of 5 mcg or 10 mcg, depending on which dose is prescribed. It is given twice a day as a subcutaneous injection (like insulin) within sixty minutes of eating breakfast and dinner.

GLP-1 hormone is structurally similar to glucagon but acts very differently. Whereas glucagon from the alpha cells of the pancreas causes the release of stored glucose from the liver to prevent low blood sugar, GLP-1 hormone

1. increases insulin secretion, but only when glucose is elevated (e.g., after meals);

2. suppresses inappropriate glucagon secretion (a problem in type 2 diabetes);

3. promotes a feeling of satiety, which may decrease food intake; and

4. slows gastric emptying, thus decreasing the spike of postprandial blood sugar (another problem in type 2 diabetes).

The most common side effect is nausea, which decreases over time. Byetta pens should be stored in the original carton (protected from the light) and in the refrigerator. Once in use, the pen should be refrigerated or kept cold, but never frozen. After thirty days, the pen should be thrown away even if it still contains medication. The pen needles should be attached right before use and properly discarded after use. Leaving needles on the pen may cause leaking or air bubbles.

The newest incretin hormone GLP-1 is Victoza (liraglutide), made by Novo Nordisk and approved by the FDA in January 2010. It also comes in an injectable pen form, like Byetta, but is given only once a day and has fewer side effects. If nausea is present, it goes away sooner. Both Byetta and Victoza can lead to pancreatitis, an inflammation of the pancreas that is painful and may be life threatening. They should not be prescribed for you if you have had pancreatitis, gallstones, a history of alcoholism, or high triglyceride levels, because these conditions make you more likely to develop pancreatitis.

How to Dispose of Medication Safely

What if your healthcare practitioner prescribes a medication but it doesn't work for you, or you have a reaction to it? What do you do with it? Many people flush unused pills, capsules, and liquid meds down the drain. The environmental impact of this practice is huge. First, it pollutes lakes and rivers as well as our drinking water. It can potentially poison wildlife, plants, and the food we eat. If we do nothing and keep it at home, it poses a poison risk for small children. Teenagers may be tempted by

What Nurses Know...

Never put medication into a container other than the one it came in from the pharmacy. In addition, keep drugs out of the sight and reach of children, and avoid taking them in front of children, because they tend to mimic adults. When giving children medication, even vitamins, avoid calling them "candy." Taking any kind of medication for adults or children is serious business.

narcotics or other drugs found in our medicine cabinets. Some people throw drugs in the trash, where others, including animals, may find them and ingest them. Also, your personal information is on the label, available for those interested in identity theft. What about giving it to friends or relatives who might be taking the same drug? This is not a good idea, because it may not really be the same medication, or the same dose, and prescribers need to be aware of what their patients are taking so they can accurately supervise the therapy. So what do you do? To help dispose of unused medication properly, the National Community Pharmacists Association has launched a "Dispose My Meds" campaign. More than eight hundred community pharmacies in forty states have already joined this effort. You can bring the drugs to a participating pharmacy, and it will send them to a medical waste disposal facility. You can also get a postage-paid envelope from the pharmacy so you can mail them yourself without leaving home. This includes any unused drugs, not just ones for diabetes. Go to www.disposemymeds. org for more details on the consequences of improper disposal of medication and to find a participating pharmacy near where you live or work. I have directions to the one closest to me posted on my refrigerator.

New Diabetes Medications Coming

As I write this section, I think about the advertisements for Windows 7 and want to say this or that innovation was my idea. Maybe some of you will want to claim a few for yourself. There are a lot of hassles with the treatment of diabetes and a lot of things can be improved to make life easier. However, diabetes management has come a long way in just the last fifteen to twenty years. As far as I'm concerned, the sky is the limit. Until we have a cure for both type 1 and type 2, let us celebrate the research that has brought and will continue to bring us easier and better ways to control blood glucose.

HOW A NEW DRUG OR PRODUCT GETS APPROVED

With almost twenty-four million people in the United States with diabetes, this is big business. Pharmaceutical and manufacturing companies take this target consumer population very seriously. Scores of new antidiabetic drugs, including new insulins and unique deliveries of such medication, as well as treatments for diabetic complications, are under investigation as you read this book. Many never come on the market, such as a nasal insulin from 10 years ago. Some take decades, such as the now-promising inhaled insulin. Some, after considerable experimentation, receive FDA approval only to be recalled because of adverse reactions, as was the case with the first TZD on the market, Rezulin. The process from development to availability involves many phases, some of which involve healthy individuals as well as those who have the disease.

Before conducting investigational trials with human subjects, scientists research new treatments in test tubes and experiment on animals, usually mice or rats, to test hypotheses about the potential use of this or that chemical combination. If they discover a promising chemical compound to treat any number of potential causes of a disease or its complications, they refine the process and then may move on to larger animals. After more refinement as to dosage, timing, method of delivery, safety, and side effect profiles, they may start clinical trials using human subjects. Phase I trials use small numbers of healthy, paid adult volunteers of both genders and most races so researchers can test the effects of an experimental drug or treatment to further refine safety, dose range, and side effects and to evaluate whether there are unintended consequences in humans, such as liver, kidney, or other potential problems. The subjects are evaluated often and are taken off the protocols if any negative reactions occur.

If all goes well in Phase I, the drug or treatment goes into Phase II testing. This usually occurs in a few research medical centers and involves a small number of clients with the disease, in this case, type 1 or type 2 diabetes. These paid volunteers must meet certain criteria. They usually receive free exams, medical care, and experimental medication or treatment to get a better drug or treatment profile and to see whether the experimental treatment works as intended in the human subjects for which it was developed. A further refinement of safety issues and dosage also occurs. This may take weeks or months, but in the end the drug or treatment is either ready for Phase III or it is scrapped or returned to the drawing board. The drugs or treatments that get to Phase III are tested in double- or triple-blind clinical trials at medical centers across the country and

What Nurses Know ...

The placebo effect occurs when the client expects something to happen and it does, even though the client was not on the real medication.

worldwide involving large numbers of volunteers for which the experimental drug or treatment was intended. The subjects are divided into a control group, which may be given a placebo or current therapy, and an experimental group, which receives the item to be tested. This phase compares the experimental treatment with currently available treatments and/or placebo. To prevent the placebo effect the study has a double-blind control, in which neither the volunteers nor those conducting the experiment knows who is receiving either the investigational therapy or a placebo.

Everything is numbered, and records are evaluated by a third party not involved in the actual experiment. Volunteers receive frequent free medical care, treatment, and instructions; records are kept; and the length of the trial is variable, from weeks to months to years. Volunteers may be lost to follow-up or taken off the protocol because of unforeseen occurrences that may or may not have anything to do with the experimental treatment. However, the trial subject numbers are so large that minor subject loss really does not alter the data. Only after all of the data from animal studies through Phase III are completed is a new drug application submitted to the FDA. The FDA evaluates the drug and all of the data submitted and either approves it, approves it provisionally, or rejects it. At any time along this path an idea may be stopped, reformulated, or continued. Once an experimental drug or treatment has been FDA approved it enters Phase IV, in which it can be prescribed to individuals fitting the criteria for which it was designed. At this point, prescribers are still submitting data on side effects and other information from the clients using this newly approved drug. This phase may go on for years and may lead to a drug being taken off the market if there are reports to the FDA of significant adverse reactions, such as with Rezulin, which caused liver damage. Another reason a drug may be taken off the market is if the manufacturer decides it is not selling well. That is what happened to the first inhaled insulin, Exubera.

FOUR PHASES OF INVESTIGATIONAL DRUG STUDIES

Phase I

Small numbers of healthy volunteers (as opposed to volunteers afflicted with the disease or ailment that the drug is meant to treat). Purpose is to determine the optimal dosage and pharmacokinetics of the drug (absorption, distribution, metabolism, excretion). Tests are performed.

Phase II

Small numbers of volunteers who have the disease or ailment that the drug is designed to diagnose or treat. Participants are monitored for drug effectiveness and side effect. If there are none, testing may proceed to Phase III.

Phase III

This phase involves a large numbers of patients at medical research centers. Large numbers provide information about frequent or rare adverse effects that have been identified in Phase II. Placebos are used to prevent bias. The study is conducted in blinded form so the investigator does not know which group has the actual drug being tested.

New Drug Application

At this point, the FDA reviews all results the company submits in the new drug application. If approved, the company is free to market the drug exclusively.

Phase IV

Postmarketing studies are voluntarily conducted to gain further proof of therapeutic effects of new drug. (When drugs are used in the general population sometimes severe adverse effects show up.)

From *The Nurse's Guide to Teaching Diabetes Self-Management* by Rita Girouard Mertig, reproduced with permission from Springer Publishing Company, LLC, New York, NY.

Volunteering to be a clinical trial participant can significantly impact the course of treatment for diabetes or any other disease or condition. Disease-free individuals are usually recruited for Phase I trials, and those with the disease are recruited for Phases II and III. Most clients are involved in Phase III. There is a detailed informed consent involved that does not bind the volunteer to remain in the study. If you would like to learn more about new and ongoing clinical trials and participant criteria, visit the National Institute of Diabetes and Digestive and Kidney Diseases home page at www2.niddk.nih.gov/ and click on "Clinical Trials." You can also check out www.clinicaltrials.gov to find clinical trials by location and condition being studied.

Now for the fun part: to answer your questions about what you can expect in the future and when. The following list of drugs currently in clinical trials was compiled by Tracey Neithercott at http://forecast.diabetes.org/magazine/only-online/diabetes-meds-horizon.

- A medication in the DPP-4 inhibitor class (e.g., Januvia and Onglyxa) that helps the body lower too-high blood glucose levels in people with type 2 diabetes.
  Stage of development: Completed Phase III; manufacturer Novartis Pharmaceuticals has submitted the drug, vildagliptin (Galvus), to the FDA for approval.
- A once-weekly version of the injectable type 2 medication exenatide (Byetta).
  Stage of development: Completed Phase III; manufacturers Amylin Pharmaceuticals, Eli Lilly, and Alkermes have submitted the drug for review by the FDA.
- A medication that alters the genes believed to cause insulin resistance in people with type 2 diabetes.
  Stage of development: Currently known as MBX-102, Johnson & Johnson's drug is undergoing Phase II clinical trials.
- Four inhaled insulins for people with type 1 diabetes.

Stage of development: Afresa has completed Phase III. An application has been submitted to the FDA by manufacturer MannKind Corp.

- A yet-unnamed product produced by MicroDose Therapeutx has wrapped up its Phase I clinical trial.
- Alveair (produced by Coremed Inc.) and a yet-unnamed product made by Baxter are both in Phase I trials.
- Two insulin skin patches for people with type 1 or type 2 diabetes.

  Stage of development: Altea Therapeutics' product, currently known as AT1391, is undergoing Phase I and II clinical trials for both types of diabetes.

- Another patch, created by Dermisonics, is in Phase I trials.
- Three insulin nasal sprays for people with type 1 or type 2 diabetes.

  Stage of development: An unnamed spray developed by MDRNA Inc. and Nasulin, developed by CPEX Pharmaceuticals, are both in Phase II trials.

- An exenatide nasal spray from Amylin Pharmaceuticals and MDRNA is in Phase II trials.

What Nurses Know...

The reason that insulin and other medications must be given by injection instead of in pill form is that the stomach acids will destroy the drug before it gets absorbed. Oral insulin has been a dream for many years, but first a developer must formulate the medication so that it can withstand the destruction of the stomach acids and get to the small intestines for absorption into the blood.

What Nurses Know...

If you want to check on the status of a particular drug on the Web, or simply see what is new or under investigation, be sure to put the current year next to your search term. This will move current information to the top of the list with this date.

- Four oral insulin medications for people with type 1 or 2 diabetes.
  Stage of development: An unnamed drug produced by Generex Biotechnology is in Phase III clinical trials.
- Emisphere Technologies is conducting Phase I and II trials on its yet-unnamed product.
- Intesulin (by Coremed) and VIAtab (by Biodel) are both in Phase I trials.
- A vaccine to prevent type 1 diabetes.
  Stage of development: The vaccine, named Diamyd and produced by Diamyd Medical, is in Phase III trials.

One more new category of drugs in late-stage clinical trials I found on WebMD is the SGLT2 molecule (sodium-glucose cotransporter) inhibitor. Two drugs in this drug class are dapgliflozin, developed by Bristol-Myers Squibb and AstraZenica, and canagliflozin, developed by Johnson & Johnson. These drugs are being studied in type 2 diabetics on metformin without normalizing their blood glucose levels. They could also be given with other oral diabetes meds. They work by inhibiting the SGLT2 in the kidney tubules that causes reabsorption of sugar and sodium that otherwise would be excreted in the urine. The result is that more sugar and sodium are excreted, resulting in lower blood

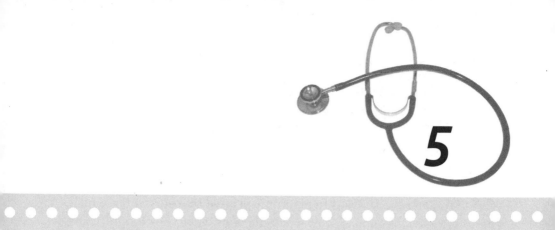

Glucose Monitoring: What Do I Do With the Results?

I test my blood sugar every morning and it is usually 180 to 200. I know that is too high, but what should I do about it? KENNY

I have type 1 diabetes and test my blood sugar before meals and at bedtime. Sometimes the numbers are around 100, where they should be. Other times they are way too high or way too low and I feel like fainting. I don't know how to fix the numbers when they are not where they should be. IRENE

The confusion and frustration both Kenny and Irene are experiencing are common for anyone who is monitoring blood glucose levels without the understanding of why the numbers may be too high or too low and what should be done about it. Until I began to figure this out for myself, all I wanted to do was throw my meter out a window, especially when the reading was high. In this chapter I explain what affects blood sugar and offer some suggestions as to how to get those numbers where you want them to be.

The bottom line with diabetes treatment is attaining near-normal blood sugars while minimizing low-glucose episodes. Several research studies, including the Diabetes Control and Complications Trial, which focused on people with type 1 diabetes, and the United Kingdom Prospective Diabetes Study, which studied individuals with type 2 diabetes, have shown significant prevention or delay of chronic complications related to high glucose levels as a result of tight control of blood sugars.

The American Diabetes Association (ADA) currently recommends the following goals for blood sugar control for both type 1 and type 2 diabetes:

Fasting	70-99 mg/dl
Before meals	70-130 mg/dl
Peak: 1 to 2 hours after meal	< 180 mg/dl
Hemoglobin A1c	< 7.0%

People without diabetes have a hemoglobin A1c of 4.0%-6.0%. A1c is a measurement of the percentage of glycosylation the average hemoglobin molecule experiences (i.e., how sugared it is) over a period of two to three months as it floats in blood containing glucose. Glucose of varying amounts is present in the blood and "sticks" to hemoglobin. Red blood cells, which contain the hemoglobin, live for about one hundred twenty days, so the glycosylated hemoglobin of these cells represents an average blood glucose level during this time period.

As you can see in the table below, the higher the A1c, the higher the average blood glucose. Therefore, following nutritional recommendations the week before you make an office visit to your healthcare provider really does not affect the results. The ADA also recommends that glycemic goals be individualized, especially with children, elderly persons, and people who are pregnant or who have frequent and severe low blood sugars. Glucose readings after meals may be particularly difficult to control if you are not giving yourself insulin, thus causing a higher A1c

CORRELATION BETWEEN A1C LEVEL AND AVERAGE PLASMA
GLUCOSE LEVELS ON MULTIPLE TESTING OVER 2 TO 3 MONTHS

A1c (%)	Meaning	Mean plasma glucose	
		mg/dl	mmol/l
5	Normal	97	5.4
6	Good	126	7.0
7	OK	154	8.6
8	Fair	183	10.2
9	Poor	212	11.8
10	Poor	240	13.4
11	High risk	269	14.9
12	Very high risk	298	16.5

mg/dl = milligrams per deciliters   mmol/l = milliosmols per liter

From *Diabetes Care*, Vol. 33, 2010; S11–S61 Reprinted and modified with permission from the American Diabetes Association. © 2010 American Diabetes Association.

average. In addition, frequent   low blood sugars may cancel out high blood sugars, thus lowering the A1c average and creating an artificially appropriate-looking percentage. This is an important point to remember. For example, prior to using an insulin pump, my A1cs were usually between 5% and 6%. However, I had frequent high and low blood sugars and my lows, especially during the night, were more significant. My seemingly great glycemic control actually indicated that I rode the blood sugar roller coaster most of the time. Since I have been using an insulin pump, my hypoglycemic episodes are very infrequent, so any high blood sugars are more noticeable. Thus, my A1cs, usually between 6.8% and 7.4%, are a truer reflection of my glycemic control.

In 2003, the ADA decreased guidelines for normal fasting blood sugar from the 1997 guidelines of 70 to 110 mg/dl to 70 to 99 mg/dl. This increased the span for impaired glucose tolerance or prediabetes from 110 to 125 mg/dl to 100 to 125 mg/dl. The purpose of both changes is to alert more people and their healthcare providers to the potential damage that can occur prior to the official diagnosis of diabetes at a blood sugar of 126 mg/dl. The hope is that this will be a wake-up call for anyone in this category to modify his or her lifestyle and get serious about weight loss, if needed, which should prevent or delay the onset of type 2 diabetes.

Hyperglycemia

Technically, higher than normal blood sugar is defined as anything above the levels given at the beginning of this chapter. The glucose levels depend on the timing of food intake from fasting and preprandial levels to one to two hours after meals. Most of us with diabetes have no symptoms until blood sugar approaches 250 mg/dl. This is an important point to remember if you do not routinely monitor your glucose levels. The most common symptoms of high blood sugar include the following:

- Frequent urination of very dilute urine (almost no color)
- Thirst from the loss of body fluids in the urine
- Hunger for simple sugars
  Other symptoms may include the following:
- Headache, sleepiness, difficulty concentrating
- Blurred vision from the glucose concentration in the eye fluids
- Dry or flushed skin from dehydration
- General malaise (feeling bad)

These symptoms may be so common in older people that they may think they are a normal part of aging. When illness, even the common cold, or other stressors increase blood sugars to 400 mg/ dl and higher, *ketoacidosis* (the by-product from burning fat) can occur. When the body does not have enough insulin to move glucose into cells for energy, the cells turn to fat to provide needed fuel. The metabolism of fat produces fatty acids and ketones that accumulate in the blood and affect the brain, producing the symptoms just listed. The kidneys try to eliminate ketones and glucose, giving rise to *ketonuria* and *glucosuria*. Testing urine for ketones with a dip stick for this purpose is confirmation that ketoacidosis is occurring. Other symptoms of this very danger-ous condition include:

- Shortness of breath
- Fruity smelling breath (like the acetone of nail polish remover)
- Nausea and vomiting

If diabetic ketoacidosis persists, the person may lapse into a coma. The blood sugar level that produces a coma is very indi-vidualized and can be anywhere from 600 mg/dl to 1,500 mg/dl or higher. This condition occurs mostly with type 1 diabetes and is caused by omitting an insulin dose, eating excessive amounts of carbohydrates, illness, and some medications. However, these same conditions, if severe enough, can over-whelm the ability of the pancreas of those of you with type 2 diabetes to respond to oral agents with an increased produc-tion of insulin. When this happens, even a person with type 2 diabetes can become ketotic. Do not assume that just because you have type 2 diabetes you cannot develop ketoacidosis. On the other hand, when ketones are *not* present in an uncon-scious person with type 2 diabetes, the resulting condition is called *hyperosmolar nonketosis*. This may happen to an elderly person who lapses into a coma from the severe dehydration caused by hyperglycemia. What all of us with diabetes need to realize is that the choice to pay attention to blood sugars may become a life-or-death decision.

FACTORS THAT RAISE BLOOD SUGAR

Many factors affect blood sugar by decreasing the effective-ness of insulin or by increasing the need for insulin. Be aware that physical stress, such as a heart attack, a stroke, trauma, pain, surgery, or infection, increases blood sugar by increasing stress hormones such as epinephrine and norepinephrine. This reaction represents the old fight-or-flight instinct we inherited from our prehistoric ancestors. We no longer have to fight the saber-toothed tiger or flee the woolly mammoth, but our adrenal glands secrete adrenalin and the other stress hormones anyway.

What we need in order to fight or flee is sufficient blood pressure (arteries constrict), increased cardiac output (heart rate increases), sufficient oxygen to hook onto each red cell being pumped out (respiratory rate increases and lung breathing tubes dilate), *and* extra glucose to fuel our brain to think and our muscles to move. Under the influence of stress hormones, stored glucose is dumped into the bloodstream by the liver and skeletal muscles. During times of physical stress, all of us with diabetes need more insulin, even if we are not eating. If you have type 2 diabetes and use oral medication to control blood sugars, you may need rapid-acting insulin injections during times of stress or crisis.

If you are hospitalized, expect nurses to test or ask you to monitor your blood glucose levels at least before meals and at bedtime even if you do not do this at home. Your healthcare practitioner will write an order stating how often this should be done and what to do about the results, from nothing to giving an injection of insulin if blood glucose exceeds 180 mg/dl or higher. Inadequate blood glucose control during hospitalization puts one at risk for infection and poor wound healing. The fear of low blood glucose may be what limits how often your medical provider orders glucose monitoring and/or insulin injections. Testing blood sugars every four hours, however, would prove that hypoglycemia does not occur if you have insulin-resistant type 2 diabetes because you become even more insulin resistant when stress hormones are released in your body. The same hormonal reaction occurs, of course, with the psychological stressors of fear, anxiety, depression, anger, and so forth. These reactions to hospitalization or other emotional stress only add to the increase of blood sugar from physical stress.

There are several medications that also increase cellular insulin resistance or that block the action of insulin. The most common is prednisone or any corticosteroid given to control the inflammatory process. If you are dealing with severe asthma; rheumatoid arthritis; systemic lupus erythematosis (SLE); or a skin, blood, or anxiety-related condition you may be taking a corticosteroid. Even a corticosteroid injected into the spine or a painful joint, or given as eye drops, can elevate blood sugar for the duration of the action of this medication if you have diabetes. Other problematic hormones that can raise blood sugar include thyroid medication; growth hormones; the body's own estrogen, either as part of the menstrual cycle or through hormonal replacement taken after menopause, and several placental hormones that increase in the second half of pregnancy. Anyone not able to increase production of insulin to counter these insulin antagonists will develop hyperglycemia. Other drugs that may increase the need for insulin include some diuretics, such as hydrochlorothiazide, Lasix, and Bumex, and large doses of caffeine (ten or more cups per day). According to Gary Scheiner, who wrote the book *Think Like a Pancreas*, weight gain itself increases insulin resistance, as does excessive sleep.

Hypoglycemia

Anyone with diabetes, especially people who are taking insulin or pills to increase their production of insulin, can experience low blood sugar. If the intake of carbohydrates does not match the amount of insulin injected or produced by the pancreas as a result of an oral sulfonylurea (see Chapter 4 for list of pertinent medications), blood sugar will drop. Everyone has his or her own reaction to hypoglycemia; however, most of us experience some of the following symptoms:

- Tremors, shakiness, or jerky movements
- Sweating, pale, moist skin
- Dizziness, feelings of being faint, headache
- Excessive hunger, especially for carbohydrates
- Sudden, atypical change in behavior, mood swings, erratic behavior

- Tingling or numbness around the mouth or tongue
- Difficulty paying attention, confusion
- Visual disturbances, difficulty reading, dilated pupils
- Increased heart and respiratory rates
- Seizures and possibly coma

As you can see, some of these symptoms sound very similar to those of hyperglycemia. It is, therefore, important to confirm these symptoms with glucose monitoring so that the meaning is clear. Because the need to treat low blood sugar is fairly immediate to prevent possible brain cell damage, when in doubt, eat. Follow the "rule of 15" (fifteen grams of carbohydrates and wait fifteen minutes). If your blood sugar is not at least 80 mg/dl, repeat. You need to do a blood test to prevent overtreating an episode of low blood sugar. Sometimes, however, you realize that you have given yourself insulin or taken a pill and then not eaten or exercised before eating, so you know that the symptoms are probably related to hypoglycemia.

Treatments for low blood sugar include a half cup (four ounces) of unsweetened orange juice, five to six hard candies (not sugar free), three to four glucose tablets, or a packet of glucose gel. The last two items can be found over the counter in most drugstores and should be carried at all time by anyone prone to hypoglycemia, including anyone on insulin, regardless of whether you have type 1 or type 2 diabetes. The following are other suggestions to treat low blood sugar: (each item equals about ten to fifteen grams of carbohydrate)

Food Item	Amount
Sugar packets	2 to 3
Fruit juice	1/2 cup (4 oz)
Soda (not diet)	1/2 cup (4 oz)
Hard candy	3 to 5 pieces
Sugar or honey	4 teaspoons
Glucose tablets	3 to 4
Glucose gel packets	1 packet

Factors That Decrease Blood Sugar

In Chapter 3 I provided an explanation of how increased physical activity, including sexual activity, improves cellular insulin
sensitivity and decreases insulin needs, perhaps for hours. If you
don't decrease the amount of insulin injected or eat more carbohydrates, hypoglycemia may result. In the same fashion, the
amount of carbohydrates, both simple and complex, must match
the amount of insulin secreted by the pancreas or given by injection or pump. If you are taking a rapid-acting insulin analogs,
such as Humalog, Novalog, or Apidra, by injection or pump, you
can wait until a meal is served to decide how many carbs you plan
to eat (see the "Carbohydrate Counting" section in Chapter 2) and
then deliver an appropriate dose of insulin. If you are taking a
rapid-acting secretagogue, such as Prandin or Starlix, with each
meal, you can omit taking it if skipping a meal or if no or very few
carbohydrate-containing foods are consumed. The problem of
needing to eat carbohydrate-containing foods occurs when you
have injected intermediate-acting insulin in the morning, which
will peak around lunchtime, or have taken a long-acting secretagogue (any of the sulfonylureas) with breakfast, which will
increase the amount of insulin secreted by the pancreas all day
long. If the carbs do not match the insulin, low blood sugar may
result. In the circumstances just described, you must eat meals
on time and provide a similar number of carbohydrate grams at
each of these meals to keep glucose levels from going too low—or
too high, for that matter.

Drugs that often decrease blood sugar include beta blockers for hypertension or arrhythmias, MAO (monamine oxidase)
inhibitors for depression, nicotine patches, and Ritalin. Giving
your healthcare practitioner a good medication history, including over-the-counter and illegal drugs you have ingested, may
unearth the cause of unexpected hypoglycemia. Alcohol also
lowers blood sugar and should always be consumed with food.
If a significant drop in blood sugar occurs after drinking an
alcoholic beverage, the liver may not be able to respond to the

glucagon secreted by the alpha cells of the pancreas, resulting in no stored glucose being released. This can become a dangerous situation. In *Think Like a Pancreas* Scheiner listed other factors that can potentially lower blood sugar, including excessive heat and humidity (especially while exercising); high altitudes; and

Factors That Increase Blood Sugar	Factors That Decrease Blood Sugar
Skipping antidiabetic medication	Too much antidiabetic medication
Overeating, especially carbs	Skipping a meal after taking medication
Significant weight gain	Significant weight loss
Decreased physical activity	Increased physical activity (even several hours later)
Medication	
Corticosteroids	Medications
Thyroid supplements	Beta blockers
Diuretics	MAO inhibitors
Caffeine (high doses)	Nicotine patch
Niacin (high doses)	Ritalin
Hormones	Alcohol
Stress hormones (adrenaline)	
Growth hormones	
Cortisol	
Pregnancy hormones	Pregnancy (1st trimester)
(2nd & 3rd trimesters)	
Hormones during menses	
Estrogen	Stress management
Emotions	
Anger	Other
Depression	Heat and humidity
Fear	High altitude
Panic	Intense brain activity
	New or unusual surroundings
Other	Socializing
Excessive sleeping	Stimulating environment

From *The Nurse's Guide to Teaching Diabetes Self-Management* by Rita Girouard Mertig, reproduced with permission from Springer Publishing Company, LLC, New York, NY 10036.

anything that may distract you from your usual routine of checking blood sugar, such as socializing, new or unusual surroundings, a stimulating environment, or intense brain work. During these times it is important to monitor blood sugars periodically and often. Set a timer, if needed, as a reminder to test. The table above is a summary of factors that increase and decrease blood glucose levels.

HYPOGLYCEMIA UNAWARENESS

Some people with type 1 diabetes may no longer sense an impending low blood sugar and may simply become unconscious when blood glucose is low enough. Because brain cells burn only glucose for energy, they stop functioning and may even die when blood glucose plummets. This very dangerous condition may affect people with long-standing type 1 diabetes, those with neuropathy that prevents the occurrence of symptoms, those who experience frequent (several times a week) and severe low blood sugars (below 40 mg/dl) as a result of tight glucose control, or those who are on beta blockers for cardiac arrhythmias or high blood pressure. Beta blockers blunt the effects of epinephrine and norepinephrine in response to low blood sugar. Some of us begin to have different symptoms as the years go by and simply fail to acknowledge them as a signal to eat something to raise blood sugar. In either case, frequent blood sugar monitoring is crucial, and eating multiple small meals becomes a necessity. Alerting others with whom you live, exercise, or work that you have diabetes is essential. You will need to get a prescription for a glucagon kit to use in case of an emergency, such as a coma or an inability to swallow juice caused by very low blood sugar. This prescription should indicate the dose of glucagon for the person for whom it was prescribed (a full dose for children age twelve and older and adults). Injected glucagon causes the liver to release stored glycogen (glucose), which should raise blood sugar within ten to fifteen minutes, enough so you can eat or drink something. Having this glucagon kit on hand and teaching others to administer the injection may become a lifesaving measure for you. Take a look at a good video by Eli Lilly and Company, a maker of glucagon, on how to administer this hormone at www.humalog.com. You and a friend, coworker, or family member should watch this video periodically to refresh your memory. When your current prescription for glucagon expires, use it for practice.

THE BLOOD GLUCOSE-SLEEP CONNECTION

In Chapter 2 I discussed the connection between inadequate sleep and obesity. People who are tired usually eat more and exercise less, causing a rise in glucose levels at night, especially if you eat before you go to bed. High blood sugars cause your kidneys to try to excrete this sugar and, with it, water. This wakes you up because you need to empty your bladder perhaps more than once during the night, thus limiting the amount of sound sleep you get. There is also some evidence that sleep deprivation can cause insulin resistance and give rise to prediabetes.

What about low blood sugar during the night? Most people on insulin have experienced this and report a variety of different symptoms than those they feel during the day. For this reason it is sometimes difficult to recognize and thus treat. Symptoms range from numbness and tingling of the lips and tongue; heart palpitations; and, if you sit up, confusion as to where you are (you don't recognize your own bedroom, even with a night light on), what your fingers are feeling (nightclothes, sheets, hands, face) and the frightening feeling that something is terribly wrong. Unfortunately, you don't have enough sugar for your brain to process the information your senses are giving it. Prior to getting my insulin pump, I experienced many nighttime lows. I would usually wake up from a recurrent nightmare sweating, confused, and frightened. Sometimes I didn't even realize the lump next to me as my husband who could, if I woke him, provide me with the help I needed. Needless to say, he saved my life and my brain cells on many occasions. For several years neither of us routinely got the sleep we needed. With the insulin pump that rarely happens.

What Nurses Know . . .

Avoid eating anything within a couple of hours of bedtime so its absorption and thus effect on blood sugar can be noted. Check your blood glucose level before you go to bed.

If it is over 200 mg/dl, take the corrective amount of insulin, if prescribed, or note this on your log so you will understand why your blood sugar is high the next morning. Then troubleshoot for why this happened, or ask your healthcare practitioner for help.

If it is below 80 mg/dl, eat something with a carb value of fifteen grams, such as a piece of fruit.

Blood Glucose Monitoring

There are many blood glucose meters on the market that rely on electrophoresis to read blood sugar. Most require a drop of blood from the finger; however, alternative sites, such as the forearm or the area of the palm below the thumb, may be used with certain types of meters. The area tested should be washed with warm water and soap; this will provide a clean surface that is free of food residue and increase the blood supply to the area. To increase the size of the drop of blood, massage the area, let the arm hang down, and/or milk the finger. To ensure accuracy, follow the manufacturer's direction as to coding the meter with each package of strips, if needed. Strips must be protected from heat and humidity. Periodic testing of strips and meter with the appropriate control solution may be necessary, especially if the glucose reading is in question. When in doubt, throw the package of strips, out. If a new package of strips does not solve the problem, call the help line number on the back of the meter. Most companies will help troubleshoot problems and/or send a replacement meter. There are lancing devices and lancets to fit everyone's coordination ability and skin depth, so you should experiment with others if the one that came with your meter is not satisfactory. Meters today require a very small drop of blood. The resource guide provided by the ADA at http://forecast.diabetes.org/magazine/features/consumer-guide-2010 provides information and comparisons for meters, strips, lancing devices, lancets, syringes, and many other supplies. Another good source to help you evaluate the particulars of meters, including A1c meters and kits, is www.mendosa.com/meters.htm.

Frequent blood sugar monitoring is recommended for both type 1 and type 2 clients. I am frequently asked how often to test, and my answer is "Whenever you need the information."

RULES TO FOLLOW FOR GLYCEMIC CONTROL

1. Carry a blood glucose meter and supplies at all times.
2. Test your blood sugar often, especially before eating; taking diabetes medication that will increase the amount of insulin in the blood; going to bed; or experiencing physical or emotional stress, including physical activity.
3. If using intermediate-acting insulin or a long-acting secretagogue, eat on a preset schedule with a predetermined amount of carbohydrates.
4. Take rapid-acting insulin or a short-acting secretagogue immediately before eating a meal with carbohydrates.
5. If hypoglycemia is a potential problem, always carry fast-acting glucose, such as gels or tablets, which are available at drugstores.
6. Always carry extra supplies needed to correct potential high blood sugar, such as extra insulin and syringes, even if you are using an insulin pump, and other antidiabetic medication, if prescribed.
7. Check expiration dates and protect supplies from extremes of heat and cold.

From *The Nurse's Guide to Teaching Diabetes Self-Management* by Rita Girouard Mertig, reproduced with permission from Springer Publishing Company, LLC, New York, NY 10036.

With all of the devices available today, it is inconceivable to me that anyone would persist in wondering what his or her blood sugar is. If you feel bad or odd, it is a simple procedure to rule in or rule out blood sugar as a cause. For a long time, insurance companies did not cover glucose strips (the expensive part of testing blood sugars) for individuals with type 2 diabetes unless they were on insulin—sort of a penny-wise and pound-foolish approach. Today, several states have passed laws that mandate that insurance companies cover meters, strips, lancing devices, and lancets, as well as diabetes education, for anyone diagnosed with diabetes. Many physicians still do not ask their type 2 patients to test blood sugar or, if they do, the testing is very sporadic. In order to understand how food and physical activity affects each individual, you must test your blood sugar. Doing lab work only at a doctor's office visit is really too little, too late. Living with a blood sugar level in the 200s or higher will cause tissue damage. The sooner hyperglycemia is discovered and treated, the less damage is done.

Now here is the big question: What should you do with the glucose monitor numbers? Currently there are many options, from low-tech lifestyle changes like omitting or decreasing the amount of certain foods or increasing physical activity, to changing medication regimens, including administration of insulin via syringe or pump. Checking your blood sugar one to two hours after eating pizza or taking a thirty-minute walk will be more convincing to you than anything you can read or hear from your healthcare provider. The increased blood sugar from eating excessive amounts of carbohydrates or the normalizing of blood sugar provided by simple exercise is very empowering. So, when should you monitor, and what do you do with the numbers?

Most of us are not convinced to change our lifestyle with scare tactics that warn of the development of chronic complications in 20 years' time. The evidence needs to be more immediate. Glycemic control improves personal well-being right now. It prevents infections and improves health. As you redefine your goals for living well on the basis of improved glycemic control

What Nurses Know...

Monitor blood sugar every day, for the following reasons:

Before giving insulin, so you can increase or decrease the amount as directed.

Before each meal and at bedtime, so you can adjust what you eat and/or any medication you take

If ≥ 180 mg/dl, eat fewer carbs or take more insulin

If ≤ 80 mg/dl, eat more carbs or take less insulin

If you have been directed to monitor your blood sugar before breakfast only and your blood glucose is routinely ≥ 180 mg/dl, follow the instructions above and test again at bedtime tomorrow.

If your bedtime blood sugar is ≥ 180 mg/dl, omit a snack and test before dinner tomorrow.

If your dinnertime blood sugar is ≥ 180 mg/dl, follow the instructions above and call your healthcare provider for further instructions.

Monitor two hours after a meal if you have made carb, insulin, or medication adjustments:

If ≥ 180 mg/dl, decrease carbs even more, increase meds, and/or call your healthcare provider

If < 180 mg/dl, you know the adjustments worked

If ≤ 100 mg/dl, cut back on the adjustments

Monitor before exercise unless you have just eaten:

If ≥ 250 mg/dl, wait until your blood sugar is lower, or take more insulin.

If ≤ 150 mg/dl, eat a fifteen-gram carbohydrate snack before exercising.

Monitor when you do not feel well to rule in or rule out whether this is related to your blood sugar level. Because illnesses do affect blood sugar, follow this advice:

If glucose is ≥ 250 mg/dl, call your healthcare provider for instructions

If glucose is 80 to 120 mg/dl, then the illness is not related and not affecting your glucose level. Repeat the test in four hours to check for changes.

If glucose is < 80 mg/dl and you feel shaky and sweaty, eat or drink fifteen grams of carbohydrates. Retest in twenty minutes.

If it is still low, eat fifteen more grams of carbohydrates.

and your health in general, you will be encouraged to continue to eat nutritiously, lose weight, increase physical activity, and follow the resulting blood sugars and periodic A1c percentages. You as well as your healthcare practitioner must also remember that no one is perfect. Blood glucose numbers are neither good nor bad; they are simply data that help us to make better choices now and in the future.

CONTINUOUS GLUCOSE MONITORS

Wouldn't it be nice to know what your blood sugar was without sticking your finger? Well, we are not there yet, but three companies so far have products that come close. They provide real-time glucose values, glucose trend information via line and bar graphs, and customized early warning alarms to warn you that your glucose levels are trending low or high so you can take action by eating (low) or giving more insulin (high) before you get into trouble. This is particularly important if your blood glucose level drops at night when you are asleep, or if you have hypoglycemia unawareness. People with type 1 and type 2 diabetes can use

them with or without an insulin pump; however, using a continuous glucose monitor (CGM) with a pump makes more sense to
me. Because insulin pumps usually have a great deal of memory,
and can remind you how much insulin is still active from your
last bolus dose based on parameters you have programmed into
your pump, it can prevent you from giving yourself more if you
have sufficient insulin on board to prevent the high trend from
going higher. More information on insulin pumps is provided in
Chapter 4.

Here is how these systems work. Continuous glucose monitoring systems (CGMSs) test blood glucose levels every five
minutes or so, depending on the system. This continues for
seventy-two hours or more, at which time the sensor must be
changed, and wirelessly transmits the information to a receiver
(cell phone size) or an insulin pump that displays the results.
(Because the CGMS transmits radio wave signals, it must be
turned off when you are flying.) A disposable sensor is inserted
via a needle, usually in the abdomen. The needle is removed,
exposing a tiny wire that measures glucose levels in the fluid
around the cells. Because a wire is involved, it must be removed
before undergoing an MRI (magnetic resonance imaging).
Because the CGMS is not testing blood directly, there is a fif-
teen-minute lag time when the sugar in the blood is moving into
this tissue fluid. A CGMS does not replace your glucose meter
because you need to periodically do a finger stick to calibrate
the system and verify a low or a high reading for accuracy. All
CGMSs require a prescription and may or may not be covered
by insurance. They are expensive and worth a call to your insurance company to see what the requirements are. If your insurer
covers a CGMS, it may require that your healthcare practitioner
justify its use for you. All CGMSs come with computer software
so you can download monitor and pump information in bar and
line graphs to e-mail to your medical provider or print and bring
with you to each office visit. This is very helpful for both of you
to troubleshoot any problems, make any treatment adjustments,
and evaluate how well you are doing.

A CGMS does not have to be used all the time. For example, I use mine when I am likely to have difficulty regulating my glucose levels, such as when I am on vacation, visiting friends or family, or any time I am not in charge of the food being served. I can fairly accurately count carbs (see my discussion of carb counting in Chapter 2), but this system gives me even more control over blood glucose levels. It warns me that I have given myself too much or too little insulin before my next manually evaluated blood sugar. Simply checking blood glucose levels even several times a day just gives a snapshot of the ups and downs of blood levels at that moment. Continuous monitoring gives you the whole video throughout the day.

The companies that currently make CGMSs include the following:

1. Metronic MiniMed, maker of the Paradigm REAL-Time continuous glucose monitor, which works with the Pardigm insulin pump and the Paradigm Revel pump with built-in CGMS, the first integrated system on the market to combine both a pump and a CGMS in one small gizmo the size of a cell phone.
2. Abbott Laboratories, which makes the FreeStyle Navigator CGMS. It transmits data wirelessly to a receiver or an insulin pump.
3. DexCom, maker of the DexCom Seven Plus, a CGMS that transmits data to a receiver.
4. Insulet, which produces the OmniPod Personal Diabetes Manager, a disposable, tubeless insulin pump with a manual glucose meter that transmits insulin delivery instructions. It can also be used with any available CGMS, such as the FreeStyle Navigator described in Item 2.
5. Animas, maker of One Touch Ping, their latest insulin pump. It must be used with a manual glucose meter.

The last two companies are both working with DexCom and its CGMS so their pumps can display and record data from the DexCom Seven Plus. Both should be available by the end of 2010.

In addition, DexCom and Insulet are in the process of developing an integrated pump/CGM OmniPod system in competition with the Metronic Revel. Metronic, on the other hand, is developing a disposable, tubeless pump like the OmniPod. Metronic also has a very sophisticated integrated system, the Veo, that automatically suspends the flow of insulin from the pump when its CGM detects hypoglycemia, an advantage for systems worn by children and individuals with hypoglycemia unawareness. So far Veo is available only in Europe, but Metronic is testing it in the United States and may soon get approval from the Food and Drug Administration.

For the techies among you there is now an app from Life Med Media compatible with the iPhone (OS 3.0 or later), iPod Touch, and iPad. At the iTunes store you can buy and download Diabetes Companion by dLife to track blood sugar, find diabetes-friendly recipes, watch videos from dLifeTV, and get answers to your diabetes questions, all for 0.99–that's right, 99 cents. Another innovation to make your life easier is the Cellnovo, the smallest insulin pump so far. It consists of a waterproof, wireless touchscreen made by Cellnovo, which can deliver insulin, adjust bolus doses, monitor glucose, track activity, access your journal, check foods, and so on. This new pump system should be available before the end of 2010. Other glucose monitoring technologies in development include some non-finger stick devices, including the nano ink tattoos that use reactive dyes and fluorescent beads that change color based on glucose changes and soft contact lenses that change color to show when glucose levels are going too high or too low. There are also gluco wristwatches with membranes on the underside that use small electric currents to draw fluid through the skin and test blood sugar that way. I have no guess as to when the last three will be available, but someday soon monitoring blood sugar may be as simple as looking in the mirror or at your watch.

Diabetes and diabetes management have become big business due to our ever increasing numbers. More and diverse companies are inventing new gadgets and vying for our business. Look for new insulin pumps, CGMSs, and systems integrating the two as well as other diabetes-related paraphernalia in the future. This should also make this equipment less expensive. Isn't competition wonderful?

The most important value of any glucose monitoring device is its impact on how you manage your diabetes. Obviously, the more data you have, the more you can analyze the information and make appropriate corrections, which should result in greater glucose control, a lower A1c percentage, and prevention of both acute and chronic complications. The better the blood sugar control, the more options you have and the more normal and fulfilling your life will be. Control of blood sugars by whatever means necessary and available can leave you free to enjoy life to the fullest. That should be the goal and the mantra for all of us with diabetes. What motivates me to eat right, move more, monitor my glucose levels, and take appropriate action, if necessary, is a slogan I repeat often. "Control will set you free"—free to enjoy family and friends and the life I want to live.

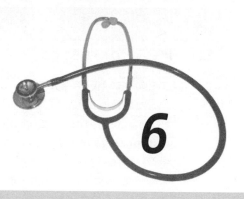

6

How Can I Prevent Complications?

My husband died of a heart attack from type 2 diabetes which he refused to take care of. My son is overweight, has type 2 diabetes and has not been taking care of himself. He recently survived a heart attack and now he is listening to his doctor. He remembers how his father died. JOAN

Most of my previous chapters have been positive and, I hope, empowering. But some of you may need to be hit in the head with a 2 × 4 or scared straight like Joan's son to get it. So here are some statistics from the Centers for Disease Control and Prevention's 2007 National Diabetes Fact Sheet (the most recent year for which data are available) that I hope will do just that.

- Adults with diabetes have heart disease death rates two to four times higher than adults without diabetes.
- The risk of stroke is two to four times higher among people with diabetes.

- Seventy-five percent of adults with diabetes have hypertension.
- Diabetes is the leading cause of new cases of blindness among adults aged twenty to seventy-four.
- Diabetes is the leading cause of kidney failure.
- About sixty to seventy percent of people with diabetes have mild to severe forms of nervous system damage. The results of such damage include impaired sensation or pain in the feet or hands, slowed digestion of food in the stomach, carpal tunnel syndrome, erectile dysfunction, or other nerve problems.
- More than sixty percent of nontraumatic lower limb amputations occur in people with diabetes.
- Young adults with diabetes have twice the risk of developing gum disease as those without diabetes.
- People with diabetes are more susceptible to many other illnesses and, once they acquire these illnesses, such as pneumonia or influenza, are more likely to have a worse prognosis than those without diabetes.

Do I have your attention yet? Now let me tell you more about each area; how to tell if something is going wrong so you can get help immediately; and, more important, how you can prevent, delay, or treat each condition.

In Chapters 2 through 5 I described in detail how to live with diabetes in order to feel well and live the life you want to live. Whether you have type 1 or type 2 diabetes, you probably don't feel bad as long as your blood glucose doesn't go above 250 mg/dl or below 60 mg/dl. However, living with a blood sugar between 200 and 250 mg/dl or higher most of the time can and does cause damage to glucose-sensitive organs even if we don't feel bad. Having an A1c of 7% means that your average blood glucose over the last two to three months is 154 mg/dl, an acceptable number considering the fact that some blood sugars were lower and some higher. But an A1c of 8% equals an average of 183 mg/dl, an A1c of 9% means 212 mg/dl, and an A1c 10% equals 240 mg/dl. The good news is that a blood glucose under 250 mg/dl doesn't usually make you sleepy or lethargic, but the bad news is that an A1c over 8% indicates fair to poor blood sugar control (see Chapter 5) and eventually causes organ damage. It may take twenty years, but unless you were seventy years old when you were diagnosed, the high blood sugars ought to concern you. You need to get as close to an A1c of 7% or below as soon as possible and do whatever it takes to keep it there.

The glucose-sensitive organs I keep talking about include the heart and all blood vessels, the brain, eyes, kidneys, nerves, skin, feet, gums, stomach and intestines, the immune system and, um...I'm still thinking. You get the picture. High blood glucose levels are like a poison to most if not all body systems and organs. This chapter will hit the high points of most complications in terms of prevention, symptoms, diagnosis, and treatment. Please remember that prevention and/or delay of complications is a lifelong goal of diabetes self-management, but it never motivated me to do what I needed to do on an hourly and daily basis. I work hard at controlling blood sugars so I can feel good today, right now, and live the kind of life I would want to live if I didn't have diabetes. With all the medications and gizmos we have today to help us normalize blood glucose levels, all we need to add is the willpower to make it happen.

Having said that, know that bad things can happened to good people. So, catching a complication as early as possible is what everyone connected to diabetes management should be looking for. Besides my endocrinologist, who is concerned with my diabetes and hypertension, I also see an ophthalmologist who specializes in diseases of the retina, a periodontal dentist who checks for gum disease, and a podiatrist who cuts my toenails and checks my feet for calluses at least once a year or more often. Diabetes is an expensive disease, but nothing takes the place of testing blood sugar levels as often as needed and correcting them when needed to live a long and healthy life. Prevention is what we all wish for but, just in case, in this chapter I cover each of the major complications so you can recognize the early warning signs and have some idea of the current treatments for each.

If you do any research on the Web for more information, please remember to put the current year after your search terms. This will put the most current information first. There is a lot of old, outdated stuff out there. One other point I'd like to make is that you may not want to read all of this chapter at once. It can be overwhelming. Start with the areas of most concern. I personally could not write this chapter from start to finish. I had to leave it and write a different chapter between topics.

Heart and Blood Vessel Disease

Heart disease is the number one killer of adults in the United States with or without diabetes. Cardiovascular complications will affect seventy-five percent of people with diabetes. These complications include atherosclerosis (fatty deposits in arteries); heart attack; hypertension; stroke; and peripheral arterial disease that can lead to decreased circulation of the feet and, potentially, an amputation. The good news is that *none* of this is inevitable, even if you do have diabetes. Risk factors for cardiovascular disease include a family history of it; smoking; uncontrolled high cholesterol, especially high low-density lipoproteins (LDL; the "bad" cholesterol), low high-density lipoproteins (HDL; the "good" cholesterol), and high triglycerides; and uncontrolled high blood pressure and high blood sugar.

CORONARY ARTERY DISEASE

The main reason heart disease, especially a heart attack, can often prove deadly is that men and women do not take symptoms seriously. The following are possible symptoms that should never be ignored:

- Anxiety or intense fear of impending doom, such as if you feel like fainting or you cannot catch your breath.
- Chest discomfort or intense pressure, like an elephant sitting on your chest or a squeezing sensation. It does not have to feel like pain.
- A cough that is persistent or wheezing, which can be a sign of heart failure, when the heart is having difficulty pumping out blood to the body and fluid backs up into the lungs.
- Dizziness or lightheadedness and even loss of consciousness from a heart attack or a dangerous heart rhythm.

- Fatigue that is not typical, especially in women.
- Nausea or unusual lack of appetite. During a heart attack, some people actually vomit. Because the heart is having difficulty pumping blood to the body, blood is not going to the stomach, so you cannot digest whatever food is in there.
- Pain in other parts of the body, such as the jaw, shoulders, arms, back, neck, or abdomen. Men more often feel pain in the left arm or jaw, whereas women experience pain in both arms or between the shoulder blades in the upper back.
- Rapid or irregular pulse, especially if accompanied by weakness, dizziness, or shortness of breath, which can mean a heart attack, heart failure, or an arrhythmia (abnormal rhythm).
- Shortness of breath, especially with any of the preceding symptoms, which can mean a heart attack or heart failure.
- Sweating, especially a cold sweat for no good reason, which could be caused by a heart attack.
- Swelling, which can mean heart failure is causing accumulated fluid, often in the feet, ankles, legs, or abdomen, as well as sudden weight gain from retained fluid.
- Weakness, often severe and unexplained, which can precede and accompany a heart attack.

Obviously any of these symptoms can be of no consequence on their own, but that should be diagnosed by medical personnel. Call 911 if you should experience any of these symptoms. Sometimes you can have a silent heart attack, with no symptoms at all. An ECG (electrocardiogram), called an EKG by some, can document that one has occurred. This should stimulate further discussion between you and your healthcare provider regarding options to increase heart-healthy activities and make a plan to prevent a second heart attack in the future.

If you have angina or chest pain, it means that you have a coronary artery (or arteries) that is (are) partially blocked, enough to restrict the flow of blood to the heart muscle. You should get a prescription for nitroglycerine tablets; carry them in a moisture-proof, opaque (blocking light) container; and keep them with you at all times. When you get chest pain, put a tablet under your tongue

What Nurses Know...

Avoid holding your breath while having a stool. This is called a valsalva maneuver and is performed by forcible exhalation against a closed airway, usually done by taking a big breath and holding it while pushing down with the abdominal muscles. This action increases the pressure inside your chest, making it harder for your heart to pump blood. It also increases overall blood pressure. If constipation is a problem, get an over-the-counter stool softener; eat more fiber-rich foods, like fresh fruit and vegetables; and drink more water. If you do have to strain, let some air out slowly, as in hissing, and make this partial breath holding brief.

because it will be absorbed very quickly by the blood vessels there. Swallowing them will prolong the absorption for thirty to sixty minutes, way too long to prevent worse consequences. If chest pain happens often you can get a prescription for a longer acting nitrate that is taken two or more times a day to keep cardiac vessels open all day, or a nitro-paste or gel patch that is taped to the body during the day. Beta blocker drugs, which reduce the effects of stress hormones on the heart, can also be used on a regular basis to prevent angina. Calcium channel blockers can also reduce the oxygen needs of the heart muscle by lowering heart rate and reducing the forcefulness of each heartbeat. A newer drug is Ranexa, a fatty acid oxidation inhibitor that gets the heart muscle to switch from burning fatty acids to using glucose for energy. Glucose metabolism requires less oxygen, so the heart can pump longer during exercise before symptoms of angina occur. There are other drugs on the horizon in this medication class. Specific cardiac aerobic exercise training can also build up collateral circulation around the partial blockage and can provide improved oxygen delivery to the affected part of the cardiac muscle.

Invasive and surgical procedures for treating angina and preventing a heart attack include angioplasty with or without stents being placed, and coronary artery bypass surgery. Angioplasty involves a balloon-tipped catheter that is threaded to the site of the narrowed or blocked cardiac artery. The balloon is then inflated to crush the fatty plaque that is causing the blockage. Often a stent is left behind to hold the artery open. Coronary artery bypass surgery is open-heart surgery done under general anesthesia that requires a hospital stay and weeks to months of rehabilitation. Usually a vein from the leg or an artery from the chest wall is sewed in place before and after the blockage, thus carrying blood around the blockage or bypassing it.

Sleep apnea, a condition in which breathing is interrupted repeatedly during sleep, can damage your heart and your brain. It is associated with a higher risk of hypertension, heart failure, and stroke. Often, people who have sleep apnea snore; may gasp and choke at night; frequently wake up exhausted because sleep was not restful; may experience headaches from brain

What Nurses Know...

No matter what treatment for angina is used, the causes of the blocked cardiac artery or arteries must be addressed to prevent a new blockage from forming. Control over cholesterol, blood pressure, and blood sugar, as well as weight loss and an increase in activity level, are essential elements of the treatment of heart disease. It goes without saying that quitting smoking and/or avoid inhaling second-hand smoke will improve your ability to survive heart disease.

cells repeatedly deprived of oxygen; and may have chest pain from periodic decreases in oxygenation, increased heart rate, and constricted blood vessels from an adrenaline surge that occurs when apnea is taking place. Losing weight, avoiding alcohol and sedatives before going to bed (because these relax throat muscles), quitting smoking, and control of blood pressure and blood sugar all help to prevent these nightly attacks. If more intense help is needed, or if sleep apnea is severe, a continuous positive airway pressure (CPAP) machine can help. This small apparatus pressurizes air and blows it through a hose attached to a mask worn at night to keep the airway open and prevent any apnic spells.

Preventing further heart damage will minimize the possibility that you will develop heart failure.

ATHEROSCLEROSIS

High cholesterol can be brought under control by decreasing saturated and trans fats in the diet and eating a diet with foods high in fiber and foods rich in monounsaturated fats and omega-3 fatty acids (see Chapter 2). Keeping blood glucose levels as close to normal as possible also helps (see Chapter 5). In addition, physical activity helps to rid the body of cholesterol

What Nurses Know...

If you think you are having a heart attack, call 911 and chew four 81-mg aspirin tablets or one 325-mg tablet, as long as you are not allergic to aspirin. Sit or lie down close to the outside door so you can be found easily by the emergency personnel, note the time by pulling out the stem of your watch to stop it or by telling the 911 operator when your symptoms started, and try to take deep breaths and stay as calm as possible.

and unhealthy fatty acids to prevent plaque buildups in arteries (atherosclerosis).

Cholesterol is a soft, waxy, blood lipid (fat). LDLs can form a fatty deposit (plaque) on the inside of artery walls that often leads to an obstruction in blood flow, causing a heart attack or stroke. HDLs, on the other hand, carry the excess cholesterol out of the body and remove the plaque deposits from arteries, so the higher your HDLs, the better. In addition to the measures described earlier, learn ways to control stress by deep breathing, putting everything in proper perspective, getting enough sleep, and finding things to laugh about every day. You can use a stress ball (at least you'll develop a great grip), or go for a walk (even if only in the hall or up and down the stairs). The table below lists cholesterol numbers you should be striving to attain.

TARGET CHOLESTEROL READINGS

	All Adults With Diabetes	Adults at High Risk for Heart Disease
Total Cholesterol	<200 mg/dl	<160 mg/dl
LDL ("bad" cholesterol)	<100 mg/dl	<70 mg/dl
HDL ("good" cholesterol)	>40 mg/dl for men >50 mg/dl for women	>60 mg/dl for men and women
Triglycerides	<150 mg/dl	<100 mg/dl

If you smoke, quit, and lose weight or maintain a healthy weight for you (get rid of fat around the waist). If these healthy lifestyle changes do not bring your cholesterol numbers under control, medication can be prescribed. You've probably seen "statin" drugs advertised on TV. They are currently the most common drugs used to decrease cholesterol levels. Other medications can also be prescribed, especially if elevated triglycerides and/or low HDLs are a problem; because they all work differently, more than one classification of drugs can be prescribed.

If triglyceride levels are normal, moderate use of alcoholic beverages can increase HDL and lower LDL. Remember that

Classification	Medication	Function	Side Effects
Statins	Crestor (rosuvastatin) Lescol (fluvastatin) Lipitor (atorvastatin) Mevacor (lovastatin) Prevachol (pravastatin) Zocor (Simvastatin)	Blocks the enzyme the liver needs to produce cholesterol, helps lower LDL cholesterol and raise HDL	↑ liver enzymes, headache, muscle aches, abdominal pain, nausea, weakness
Fibrates	Lopid (gemfibrate) TriCor (fenofibrate) TriLipix (fenofibrate)	Lowers cholesterol & triglycerides	Fever, nausea, vomiting, weakness
Bile-acid binding resins	Colestid (colestipol) Prevalite (cholestyramine) Questran (cholestyramine) Welchol (colesevelam)	Binds with bile acids in the gut & lowers total & LDL cholesterol and triglycerides	Constipation, diarrhea, flatulence, bad taste in mouth
HMG-CoA reductase inhibitor	Zetia (ezetimibe)	Reduces the absorption of cholesterol or other sterols from the gut	Abdominal pain, back pain, diarrhea, joint pain, sinusitis
High-dose niacin, vitamin B-3, or nicotonic acid	Endur-Acin Niacin SR Niacor Niaspan Nicotinex Slo-Niacin	Blocks the breakdown of fats so ↓ VLDL & cholesterol & ↑ HDL	Flushing, rash, itching, nausea, vomiting, gas, ↑ blood pressure

(Continued)

Classification	Medication	Function	Side Effects
Omega-3-acid ethyl esters	Lovaza (EPA + DHA or high-dose fish oil)	↓ Triglycerides made in liver	Burping, heartburn, nausea, back pain, rash
Combinations	Advicor (lovastatin + niacin) Pravigard (pravastatin + aspirin) Simcor (simvastatin + niacin) Trilipix (atorvastatin, simvastatin, fenofibricacid) Vytorin (ezetimibe + simvstatin)	See above	See above

Note: HMG-CoA = 3-hydroxy-3-methylglutaryl-coenzyme A; VLDL = very low-density lipoprotein; EPA = eicosapentaenoic acid; DHA = docosahexaenoic acid.

moderate drinking means no more than one drink for women or two drinks for men per day. No, you can't save up and use your accumulated number on the same day. That is called binge drinking and causes many more problems than it solves. If you don't drink, don't start now. Alcohol also raises triglycerides, which may make this plan counterproductive.

HYPERTENSION

High blood pressure is another health concern that can lead to heart disease, stroke, and peripheral artery problems. It also damages the eyes and kidneys. Risk factors for high blood pressure include a family history, membership in certain ethnic groups (African Americans and Native Americans), age (the older we are, the greater the risk), and gender (men have a greater risk until age forty-five; women catch up between age forty-five to fifty-four and then surpass men at fifty-five and beyond). These are the risk factors over which we have no control.

An unhealthy, high-salt diet; obesity; and high stress levels are factors that we can control. Those of us with diabetes are at high risk for hypertension and often develop hypertension at an earlier age than our brothers and sisters without diabetes. A diet high in saturated and trans fats causes narrowing of arteries from plaque, which increases blood pressure. A high sodium intake causes kidneys to hold onto fluid, which increases the pressure on arterial walls. As if that were not bad enough, increased stress hormones cause further constriction of arteries made stiff with fatty plaque. So, dietary changes can make a huge impact on blood pressure (see Chapter 2). The DASH Diet (Dietary Approach to Stop Hypertension) consists of low-sodium, high-potassium fruits, vegetables, and whole-grain foods. Wise food guidelines include the following:

1. Eat fresh fruits at each meal.
2. Eat one or two servings of vegetables at lunch and dinner.
3. Switch to low-fat or fat-free dairy products.
4. Eat whole-grain breads and cereals.
5. Eat one quarter cup of nuts or two tablespoons of a nut butter most days.
6. Choose lean meats (skinless chicken or turkey, lean beef, fish, boiled ham, pork tenderloin).
7. Cook using low-fat methods (baking, roasting, broiling—no butter, grilling, microwaving, steaming).
8. Add little to no salt at the table or during cooking.
9. Try herbs, herb blends, light salt, salt substitutes, and spices instead of salt.
10. Read food labels and choose foods with less than 400 mg of sodium per serving.

Physical activity can also help to lower blood pressure. Three or four 10-minute walks per day can relieve stress, relax blood vessels, and help with weight management or loss. That sounds like a win–win situation to me. If you smoke, quit, and avoid inhaling second-hand smoke. Nicotine constricts arteries and thus raises blood pressure. Also, excessive (more than one or two drinks) alcohol can increase blood pressure. The American Diabetes Association and the National Institutes of Health recommend a target blood pressure of less than 130/80. In the table that follows, please note the *and*, meaning both numbers are need to be considered ideal. The *or* means that either number is considered abnormal and in need of lowering using all means possible, including medication.

If your blood pressure goes up at the doctor's office, it could be due to "white coat hypertension." Have the nurse repeat the reading at the end of the visit.

Again, when lifestyle changes are not enough, there is always medication. Often more than one type of blood pressure medication may be needed. The above table lists the many antihypertensive medications by classification, with brief descriptions of how they lower blood pressure and their side effects:

BLOOD PRESSURE RANGES

	Systolic (top number)		Diastolic (bottom number)
Ideal normal	<120	and	<80
Prehypertension	120–139	or	80–89
Hypertension Stage 1	140–159	or	90–99
Hypertension Stage 2	160 or higher	or	100 or higher

What Nurses Know...

To get an accurate blood pressure anywhere, even at home, be sure to sit quietly for at least five minutes, with your feet on the floor and your arm flexed at the elbow, relaxed, and at the level of your heart (rest your arm on a desk or table). Check both arms and, if there is a difference, record the higher pressure.

Classification	Medication	Function	Side Effects
ACE Inhibitors	Accupril (*quinapril*) Altace (ramipril) Capoten (captopril) Coversyl, Aceon (perindopril) Gopten (trandopril) Lotensin (benzapril) Monopril (fosinopril) Prinivil (lisinopril) Vasotec (enalapril) Zestril (lisinopril)	Inhibits the enzyme that converts angiotensin I to angiotensin II, a strong blood vessel constrictor. Keeps blood vessels dilated to lower blood pressure.	Cough, ↑ blood potassium, dizziness, headache, rash, metallic taste in mouth, weakness
ARBs	Atacand (candesartan) Avalide (irbesartan) Benicar (olmesartan) Cozaar (losartan) Diovan (valsartan) Micardis (telmisartan) Teveten (*eprosartan*)	Blocks the angiotensin II receptors on blood vessels so they do not constrict.	Dizziness, hypotension, high blood potassium, headache, diarrhea, metallic taste in mouth

Beta blockers	Corgard (nadolol)
	Inderal (propranolol)
	Levetol (penbutolol)
	Lopressor
	  (metoprolol)
	Normodyne
	  (labetolol)
	Prent (acebutolol)
	Sectral (acebutolol)
	Tenomin (atenolol)
	Timolide (timolol)
	ToprolXL
	  (metoprolol)
	Viskin (pindolol)
	Zebeta (bisoprolol)
		Blocks beta receptors on blood vessels so stress hormones cannot cause them to constrict.	Diarrhea, stomach cramps, rash, nausea, vomiting, muscle cramps, headache, depression. May mask symptoms of hypoglycemia.

(*Continued*)

Classification	Medication	Function	Side Effects
Calcium channel blockers	Adalat (nifedipine) Procardia (nifedipine) Calan (verapamil) Cardene, Cardene SR (*nicardipine*) Cardizem (diltiazem) DilacorXR (diltiazem) Nimotop (*nimodipine*) Norvasc (amlodipine) Plendil (*felodipine*)	Slows the movement of calcium into the cells of the heart and blood vessel walls, which makes it easier for the heart to pump and widens blood vessels.	Constipation, nausea, rash, headache, edema, hypotension, drowsiness, dizziness
Diuretics	Hydrodiuril (hydrochlorothiaside) Bumex (bumetanide) Lasix (furosimide)	Makes kidneys excrete more water in the urine, thus ↓ blood pressure.	Fatigue, thirst, weakness, muscle cramps, hypotension
Alpha blockers	Cardura (doxazosin) Hytrin (terazosin) Minipress (prozosin)		

Note: ACE = angiotensin-converting enzyme; ARB = angiotensin receptor blocker.

What Nurses Know...

If you look at the generic names of the various antihypertensives in the table, you will notice that ACE (angiotensin-converting enzyme) inhibitors all end in -pril, ARBs (angiotensin receptor blockers) end in -sartan, beta blockers end in -olol, most calcium channel blockers end in -dipine, diuretics end in -ide, and most alpha blockers end with -zosin. This is an easy way to keep track of what kind of blood pressure medication you are taking.

Keeping track of blood pressure is important, because hypertension is often called the "silent killer." Unless it rises rapidly, it usually does not have any symptoms. If you suddenly develop any of the following symptoms, however, consider this an emergency and seek help immediately:

- Feeling confused or other neurological symptoms
- Nosebleeds
- Fatigue
- Blurred vision
- Chest pain
- Abnormal heartbeat

Of course, these symptoms could be caused by something else other than hypertension, but none of these symptoms should be ignored.

STROKE (OR BRAIN ATTACK)

There are two kinds of strokes. The rarer and more fatal kind is a *hemorrhagic stroke*, in which a brain blood vessel ruptures. Unless the aneurysm or other vessel malformation is discovered

What Nurses Know...

Avoid oral decongestant medication. It will raise your blood pressure whether or not you are taking an antihypertensive medication. The higher your blood pressure, the harder your heart has to pump to get blood out to the body. If the heart cannot get enough blood and oxygen to the kidneys, the kidneys will produce renin, which will cause constriction of blood vessels and raise blood pressure even higher.

early and removed or stented, this is not something you can usually prevent. The much more common stroke is caused by a buildup of fatty plaque in the carotid arteries, (one on each side of the neck), the main vessels that supply blood to the brain or one or more of the smaller cerebral arteries. When these vessels get blocked or significantly decreases the blood supply to a part of the brain, you have a brain attack, like a heart attack. The part of the brain without a good blood supply begins to die, as does the heart muscle in a heart attack.

Symptoms of a stroke depend on which side and which area of the brain is affected. They may include:

- one-sided muscle weakness of the face, arm, or leg;
- numbness or tingling of one side of the body;
- difficulty speaking or understanding another's speech;
- vision problems, such as double vision, decreased vision, or loss of vision; or
- dizziness, loss of balance, or trouble walking.

The narrowing or blockage of arteries in the brain can be seen using a CT (computerized tomography) scan or an MRI (magnetic resonance imaging) scan. If a clot is present, "clot-busting" drugs must be given within hours of a stroke, so calling 911 is imperative. Other treatment options include a carotid

What Nurses Know...

Warning signs of a stroke include brief lapses in brain function such as confusion, visual disturbances, and difficulties in walking and talking, often called a transient ischemic attack *(TIA).*

endarterectomy to remove the fatty plaque buildup, thus restoring blood flow to the brain if this is the problem. Another surgical procedure, a carotid stenting, consists of a tube that is inserted into the blocked or narrowed brain artery. A balloon is then inflated, breaking up the plaque, and a stent, or mesh tube, is left in place. Treatment after a stroke includes rehabilitation therapies to restore function and/or help clients learn new ways of using the parts of the body weakened by the stroke. Therapies may include physical, occupational, or speech rehabilitation, as well as psychological counseling. Prevention of future attacks include quitting smoking; avoid inhaling second-hand smoke; and controlling blood sugar, blood pressure, and cholesterol with healthy meal planning, physical activity, and medication.

PERIPHERAL ARTERIAL DISEASE

Another area of blood vessel concern includes the arteries of the legs and feet (the ones farthest from the heart). Your healthcare provider should be checking the pulses on the top of your feet and behind your inner ankle bone. One way for you to check circulation is to press on the skin over the bone on top of your foot. It should blanch, and the color should return quickly when you remove your finger or thumb. If your toenails look healthy and you have hair on your toes, tops of your feet, and lower legs, your circulation to your feet is good. Hair and nails are the first to be deprived of blood supply when circulation diminishes. Since my diagnosis with diabetes, I love looking at my hairy toes and never put polish on my toenails so I can check the circulation. Of course, if you have never had hair on your toes, use the pressing of the skin on your upper feet technique to check for circulation.

Another indication of arterial narrowing in the legs is *intermittent claudication* (cramping) of the calves, thighs, and even buttocks. This occurs when walking or exercising the legs and is promptly relieved by stopping the activity. Because the exercised

What Nurses Know...

Ways to increase blood supply to the leg muscles include carrying a cane with a seat while walking until you have leg pain. Then sit until the pain goes away, usually a few minutes. Then try to walk some more. Do this a few times during your walk. In so doing, your muscles will develop collateral circulation around the blocked or narrowed artery. As time goes on, you should be able to walk farther and farther before pain starts. This can also be done using a treadmill. Strength training exercises for calf and thigh muscles can also increase collateral circulation.

muscle cannot get enough blood supply, it cramps and causes pain that is similar to the angina pain of narrowed coronary arteries.

Medication used to increase circulation to partially blocked arteries of the legs include:

- Pletal (cilostazol), which widens the arteries that supply blood to the legs and prevents platelets from sticking together and to the plaque narrowing the artery so a clot will not completely block the artery.
- Trental (pentoxifylline), which thins the blood and makes red cells more flexible so they can maneuver around narrowed arteries.
- Plavix (clopidogrel), which helps prevent harmful blood clots that may cause heart attacks or strokes. Peripheral arterial disease increases the risk for heart attacks and strokes.

Surgical correction for intermittent claudication consists of the following options:

1. Percutaneous transluminal angioplasty, in which a balloon is used to crush the fatty plaque and dilate the blocked artery. Sometimes a stent (thin wire mesh sleeve) can be inserted to keep the vessel opened. This stent may be coated with an anti-coagulating medication to prevent clots from forming in the future.
2. Surgical bypass of the blocked artery, which can be done using one of a person's own veins or a synthetic Dacron graft so blood flow can go around the blocked area much the same way that it is done for coronary artery disease.

Poor circulation is also a by-product of nicotine, so if you smoke, *stop*, and avoid breathing in second-hand smoke. As a nurse, the worst case of circulation deficits in the feet and legs I ever saw was in a 60-year-old client who smoked and did *not* have diabetes. She eventually lost both legs and died of infection and lack of wound healing. During all of her many admissions

What Nurses Know . . .

Prevention for all cardiovascular diseases is the same. Follow the ABCs:

A1c less than 7%
Blood pressure below 130/80
Cholesterol <200 mg/dl, LDL <100 mg/dl (better yet, <70 mg/dl), HDL >40 mg/dl for men and >50 mg/dl for women (better: >60 mg/dl for everyone), triglycerides <150 mg/dl (better: <100 mg/dl)

for surgery she refused to stop smoking, even knowing that it would soon kill her.

Talk to your healthcare practitioner about taking a baby aspirin (81 mg) each day to prevent platelets from sticking to plaque in the arteries and forming a clot. Quit smoking by any and all means possible. Take prescribed medication as directed. If you can't afford your medication and generics are not available, ask your healthcare provider to refer you to any of the programs mentioned at the beginning of Chapter 4. Many pharmaceutical manufacturers provide their nongeneric meds at no or reduced cost to those who meet certain criteria. Whatever you do, do not stop taking prescription meds without talking to your healthcare professional.

Vision Problems

By far the most troublesome part of all the complications for me is fear of blindness. Having had type 1 diabetes for 25 years puts me at risk for *retinopathy*, or damage to the retina, the light-sensitive nerve tissue in the back of the eye, and other vision issues.

RETINOPATHY

Almost everyone with type 1 diabetes, and more than seventy percent of those with type 2, will eventually develop some degree of retinopathy, often, thankfully, without any loss of vision. *Nonproliferative retinopathy* is the early stage, when the tiny blood vessels that feed the retina weaken and form bulges that can leak small amounts of blood or fluid into the surrounding tissue. This can begin to happen after fifteen years or sooner with type 1 diabetes. Vision at this stage is usually not affected, but an ophthalmologist experienced with diabetic retinopathy should be checking you for progression, probably every four to six months. This can progress very slowly over many years or can rapidly deteriorate depending on control of blood sugar and blood pressure.

Proliferative retinopathy is the next stage, when fragile new blood vessels grow on the retina and out into the gel (vitreous) in the back of the eye as a result of poor oxygenation of the retina caused by high blood sugars. These blood vessels can rupture and bleed into this gel, causing burred vision or temporary blindness. If scar tissue forms on the retina, it can cause a detachment and, if not reattached soon, lead to loss of vision in that area. I recently experienced bleeding into the vitreous gel of my left eye, which caused my 20/20 eyesight in that eye to deteriorate to 20/400 (the big E on the eye chart). Over the last seven months, my body has absorbed more and more of the blood in the back of the eye, and my eyesight has improved to where I now see 20/25 in that eye without treatment.

To prevent the worst-case scenario from happening, your ophthalmologist should do a thorough exam of the retina through dilated pupils (when drops are used to open the pupils) every six months to one year, depending on the circumstances. These exams should start after five years with type 1 diabetes. Individuals with type 2 should start yearly exams as soon as possible after diagnosis because diabetes may have been present for several years.

Maintaining tight blood glucose control (A1c < 7%) and keeping blood pressure under 130/80 can help prevent the onset and progression of the retinal damage. A 2009 study showed that being on an ACE inhibitor or an ARB for hypertension can slow the development of retinopathy by seventy percent. (See the list of antihypertensive medications listed earlier in this chapter.)

Treatment of proliferative retinopathy with laser photocoagulation can zap fragile blood vessels before they bleed and reattach the retina, if needed, to preserve vision. This is an outpatient procedure and usually does not cause pain. As part of the prevention of further bleeding, my ophthalmologist recently used the laser on parts of the retina of my left eye. All I felt was some mild pressure and a few hours of blurry vision from all of the drops used before and after the procedure. I was afraid I'd move during the procedure, but the nurse held my head firmly against the band at my forehead to prevent that. If there has been extensive bleeding into the vitreous gel, a vitrectomy can be done. This is also an outpatient procedure in which the vitreous gel in the back of the eye is removed and replaced by a saline solution. Most people notice an improvement in vision and can resume reading and driving. Sometimes the body can absorb the blood if it is not continuous and the situation can resolve itself, as it did in my case.

MACULAR DEGENERATION

The *macula* is the site on the retina that focuses on central vision needed to see straight ahead for reading; driving; and doing any close work, such as knitting or needlepoint. This is different from peripheral vision, which is needed to see things on the side and also is needed for driving. Macular degeneration is often age related and familial, and it is progressive. There are two types of macular degeneration, dry and wet. Dry macular degeneration represents about ninety percent of all cases, occurs in both eyes, and progresses much more slowly, which is good because there is currently no treatment for this form. In this type, waste material deposits, called *drusen*, develop on the retina but usually do not affect vision unless they are numerous and involve the fovea, the very central area of the macula. One thing that has been shown to prevent and improve vision in age-related macula degeneration is omega-3 fatty acids. They prevent inflammatory and degenerative disease of the brain, nervous system, and retina. So eat fatty fish, such as salmon, tuna, or mackerel, twice a week, or take a fish oil supplement every day.

Wet macular degeneration, on the other hand, accounts for about 10% of cases but causes much more vision loss and progresses more rapidly. This is the type more often related to diabetes than to age and results from the leaking and hemorrhaging of the tiny new blood vessels of proliferative retinopathy mentioned earlier. If these vessels are around the macula, the leaking causes *macula edema* (i.e., wet), and central vision is threatened unless treatment begins soon. Prevention is most important, but next to that are early diagnosis and treatment with laser photocoagulation to eliminate the blood vessels that are leaking or that might in the future. Because I already have proliferative retinopathy, I listen to what my ophthalmologist dictates to his nurse as he is looking into my dilated pupils. When he says "The macula is dry," it is like music to my ears. If you are at risk for macular degeneration, ask your ophthalmologist for an Ambler Grid to take home to test for development of the condition. The lines of the grid should not be wavy or distorted. Test each eye separately. Mine is on my refrigerator so it doesn't get lost, and I see it every day. It also makes me think to test my blood sugar when I want something sweet in the freezer.

Other treatments for wet macular degeneration include a series of intraocular injections of anti-VEGF (vascular endothelial growth factor) medication such as Avastin, Lucentis, or Macugen. These injections are done in the ophthalmologist's office and usually improve vision and stabilize the eye from further vision loss. VEGF is a protein that allows the tiny blood vessels of retinopathy to grow and proliferate. By blocking the action of this protein in the eye, the tiny blood vessels shrivel up and die, thus preventing any further leakage from current vessels. However, new vessels can grow, necessitating repeat injections. A newer treatment, Ozurdex, is a sustained-released drug delivery system that releases steroids into the eye for four to six months. It is approved by the Food and Drug Administration to treat retinal veins but may soon be approved for diabetic retinopathy as well. On the horizon is another sustained-release steroid delivery system, called Iluvien. It is now awaiting Food and Drug Administration approval. This system will last for twenty-four months after injection. The vehicle that delivers the steroid is tiny and is injected via a 25 gauge needle. For comparison, insulin is injected into the fatty tissue with a 31 gauge needle, which is very tiny, and most intramuscular injections for pain or antibiotics are done with a 23 gauge needle, larger. The vehicle remains in the eye, but it is miniscule. This is a small price to pay for improved vision.

CATARACTS AND GLAUCOMA

These conditions are more common in people with diabetes and can develop at an earlier age than in people without diabetes.

What Nurses Know...

The smaller the gauge of a needle, the larger the bore, or inside diameter. This does not tell you anything about the length of the needle, just the inside diameter. For example, blood transfusions are delivered using an 18 gauge (large) needle, and insulin syringes have a 31 gauge (very small) needle.

A *cataract* is a clouding of the lens of the eye and, over time, it impairs vision. Basically, in those of us with diabetes it is caused by an excess level of blood glucose, which sticks to the lens. Today when a cataract is removed, a lens implant that can correct for vision is inserted. This implant can even correct astigmatism. In the near future it may also make the need for reading glasses obsolete.

With *glaucoma* the high fluid pressure within the eyeball can damage the optic nerve (part of the retina), which carries what you see to the brain for interpretation. Each time you have an appointment with an optometrist or ophthalmologist for an

What Nurses Know...

When cataracts are removed and you also have some form of retinopathy, the risk of a vitreous bleed is increased. The eye surgeon should look at the retina with your pupils dilated in all follow-up visits and at least every six months thereafter.

eye exam your eye pressure should be measured. Because this increase in pressure causes no symptoms until the damage is done, you should have this pressure tested at least once a year. Treatment usually consists of eye drops to lower the intraocular pressure. If this is not enough, laser treatment may be necessary to prevent loss of vision. Being proactive in getting eye exams and following through with any treatment necessary is a must, as is tight glucose and blood pressure control, to preserve vision.

Kidney Damage (Nephropathy)

The tiny blood vessels, called *capillaries*, of the nephrons, the working units of the kidney, can be damaged from excessive blood glucose levels and uncontrolled hypertension. About thirty to forty percent of people with type 1 diabetes, and twenty percent of those with type 2 diabetes, will eventually develop some kind of kidney damage. The kidneys and their nephrons filter the blood constantly to remove waste products, including metabolized drugs. They play a major role in fluid and electrolyte balance.

When your kidneys can no longer get rid of excess body fluids, blood pressure goes up and the risk of a heart attack, stroke, or eye damage increases. Because everyone with diabetes is at risk for renal disease, urine should be tested for small amounts

What Nurses Know...

Electrolytes, such as sodium, potassium, magnesium, calcium, and phosphorus, regulate our nervous system, make our muscles contract and relax, help blood to clot (calcium), and keep our bones strong (calcium, magnesium, and phosphorus).

of protein called *albumin* once a year. The condition, if the urine test $\geq$ 30, is called *microalbuminuria*. This may start to develop as early as five to ten years after diagnosis. If present, it may take another ten years or so for larger amounts of protein to appear in the urine (*proteinuria*) due to worsening damage to the nephrons. There should be no protein lost in the urine under ordinary circumstances, so proteinuria is a late sign of renal damage. Another test that should be done yearly to assess kidney function is a *blood creatinine*. Healthy kidneys should filter this waste product out of the blood. Renal insufficiency is a decreased ability of the kidneys to filter the blood. This condition may progress slowly for many years. When the nephrons can no longer get rid of wastes and excess fluid, kidney failure has occurred. At this point, dialysis—either hemodialysis or peritoneal dialysis—or kidney transplantation are the only options.

The strategies to prevent or slow the progression of kidney damage include:

1. Tight glucose control (A1c <7%)
2. Successful treatment of hypertension (< 130/80)
3. Adding an ACE inhibitor or ARB if not already prescribed for hypertension (see the list of medications for hypertension presented earlier in this chapter)
4. Limiting the use of NSAID (nonsteroidal anti-inflammatory) pain relievers, lab tests that use contrast dye, and any other medication that can damage kidneys
5. If kidneys continue to fail, limiting protein intake may be needed to decrease the stress on the nephrons.

Symptoms of kidney failure include fatigue, weakness, headaches, itchiness, nausea, vomiting, loss of appetite, foamy dark urine that is decreased in amount, and fluid retention, which can cause edema and an increase in blood pressure. Fatigue and weakness come from anemia because the failing kidneys cannot produce erythropoietin, a hormone that stimulates the bone marrow to produce red blood cells. Like insulin, this hormone can be

What Nurses Know...

The most important strategies to prevent kidney damage are tight blood sugar and blood pressure control. If kidney function is decreased, any medication that is excreted in urine may need a dosage reduction.

given by injection in the fatty tissue of the abdomen. As soon as renal failure is diagnosed, most people are placed on the kidney transplant list and dialysis is begun.

HEMODIALYSIS

This treatment to filter the blood outside the body is done in special dialysis centers and takes from three to five hours, three times per week. There is a special shunt placed in the arm or leg between an artery and a vein. The artery is hooked up to a machine that takes the blood and passes it through a dialysate solution that removes the waste products of the body's metabolism, any drugs and other products broken down by the liver, and excess water, all of which the kidneys would do if they could. The cleansed blood is returned to the body via a tube inserted in the vein part of the shunt. Many people feel very weak after this procedure because their blood pressure, which was high from excess water before the procedure, is now low. Maintaining an intact shunt is very important, because there are only a few places in the arms and legs where this shunt can be placed.

- Make sure your nurse or technician checks your access site (where the shunt is placed) before each treatment.
- Keep your access site clean at all times.

- Use your access site only for dialysis.
- Be careful not to bump or cut your access site.
- Don't let anyone put a blood pressure cuff on the arm which has your access site.
- Don't wear jewelry or tight clothes over your access site.
- Don't sleep with your arm that has the access site under your head or body.
- Don't lift heavy objects or put pressure on your arm with the access site.
- Check the pulse in your access site every day.

PERITONEAL DIALYSIS

This method of cleansing the blood is usually done by the person or a family member at home or at work after careful instruction is given. Peritoneal dialysis requires a surgically implanted catheter in the abdomen through which the dialysate or dialysis solution is delivered. This solution is hung higher than the body, which allows it to flow into the abdomen by gravity and passes through the peritoneal membrane (in the abdomen) which filters out the waste products and excess fluid from the body. The empty bag is then lowered below the body so the fluid containing the waste products can then drain out. The old bag is disconnected and discarded. This procedure is done every day and takes about thirty to sixty minutes. There are cycler type machines that can be connected and used at night. Peritoneal dialysis gives the person much more flexibility in scheduling, there are fewer dietary restrictions, and he or she often feels better because wastes and fluids are removed every day and do not build up. Infection is the number one problem with this method of dialysis. To prevent infection:

- Store supplies in a cool, clean, dry place
- Inspect each bag of solution for signs of contamination
- Find a clean, dry, well-lighted space to perform the exchanges
- Wash your hands every time you need to handle your catheter
- Clean the exit site with an antiseptic every day

- Wear a surgical mask when performing exchanges

Watch for signs of infection, such as:

- Fever
- Nausea or vomiting
- Redness or pain around the catheter
- Unusual color or cloudiness in used dialysis solution

If any of the preceding occurs, the person must call a health-care practitioner promptly so the problem can be treated.

KIDNEY TRANSPLANTATION

The ultimate remedy for kidney failure is a kidney transplant from a live donor or a person who has donated his organ when he dies. It may take awhile for a kidney to become available, so dialysis is done as a stopgap measure. Because people need only one kidney, a close family member whose HLA (human leukocyte antigen) markers match may choose to give one to the person who is in renal failure. When a person with type 1 diabetes needs a kidney, a pancreas or partial pancreatic transplantation may also be done. Although immunosuppressant drugs have come a long way in recent years in preventing rejection of the transplanted kidney, they must be taken for life, and they may cause the recipient to be unable to fight off common infections and some cancers. Prevention of kidney damage is definitely preferable.

Nerve Damage (Neuropathy)

Diseases of the nervous system affect about sixty to seventy percent of people with both type 1 and type 2 diabetes. Tight control of blood glucose (Alc < 7%) decreases the risk of nerve damage by up to sixty percent. Peripheral neuropathy affects nerves of the feet, legs, hands, and arms. Automatic neuropathy affects the nerves of the autonomic nervous system, which regulates body functions not under our conscious control. Neither of these conditions is pleasant or easily managed.

PERIPHERAL NEUROPATHY

Many people with type 2 diabetes are diagnosed when they see a healthcare practitioner for numbness, tingling, or pain, especially in the feet, that often keeps them awake at night. Obviously they have had high blood sugars for many years before nerve damage occurred. Peripheral neuropathy puts you at risk for other problems of the limbs, especially when combined with poor circulation, as with peripheral artery disease, discussed earlier in the chapter. Continuous high blood glucose levels are toxic to nerve fibers and eventually kill them. When your feet are numb, you don't feel a blister or a stone in your shoe! A wound can get infected and, if circulation is impaired, the white blood cells that fight infections and the red blood cells that help an injury heal don't get to the site. A simple blister can be the start of what may end up as an amputation.

In addition to high blood sugars, hypertension, cardiovascular problems, and high cholesterol increase your risk for developing neuropathy. These problems, if uncontrolled, result in poor circulation that deprives the nerves of oxygen. Controlling blood sugar, blood pressure, and cholesterol with or without medication are the most important things you can do to prevent neuropathy or to minimize nerve damage if it is already present. Because nicotine affects circulation, quit smoking and avoid taking in second-hand smoke.

Nerves are classified as either *sensory nerves* or *motor nerves* or serve both functions. Sensory nerves let us know when sand or a rock gets in our shoes or when we try to walk barefoot on hot cement around a pool. When they are damaged, we feel numbness; tingling, burning; and sharp, jabbing pain at, for example, the least touch of the sheets on our toes. These sensations are more noticeable at night because we are not so distracted by what is going on around us. It makes sleeping very difficult.

Motor nerves send signals to our feet and leg muscles to contract and relax as we walk, run, or jump. When they are damaged it may be difficult to raise the front of the feet, and a condition called *foot drop* develops. The muscles become weak and don't respond well to loss of balance, so falls are more probable. There is also lack of coordination and perhaps even paralysis. When muscles are not stimulated they get smaller, which increases weakness. Both sensory and motor involvement can occur in the hands as well, and writing, picking up small objects, and even turning the page of a book can become difficult. Picking up anything even slightly heavy can become impossible if weakness of the hands and forearms is involved.

The good news is if you are feeling the early signs of sensory nerve damage you can do a lot to improve this condition by controlling blood sugars and the other causes mentioned earlier. The bad news is that if you don't work at this, your sensory nerves may die and you will feel nothing in your feet. Pain is a protective mechanism that makes us remove our foot or hand from whatever caused the pain, such as a rock or a nail or a hot stove. When feet, in particular, lose sensation, an ulcer can form and, if left untreated, can become gangrenous and necessitate an amputation of one or more toes, or worse. Your healthcare practitioner

What Nurses Know . . .

Another thing besides high blood sugars that can lead to neuropathy is a decrease in vitamin B-12 absorption. The diabetes drug metformin (Glucophage) can decrease the absorption of this important vitamin. Also, as we age we lose some of the cells in the stomach that produce intrinsic factor necessary for B-12 absorption. After removal of part of the stomach because of cancer surgery or stomach reduction due to gastric bypass surgery or stomach banding for weight loss, vitamin B-12 injections may be necessary to maintain nerve cell health and to prevent anemia.

should be testing for peripheral neuropathy at every visit by using a monofilament to determine whether you feel where it touches the underside of your feet and placing a tuning fork on the knuckle of your big toe to test your vibratory sense. Vibratory sensations are the first to go before the sense of light touch as you are experiencing neuropathy.

The following are some treatments to ease the discomfort of sensory nerve damage:

- Pain relievers, such as Extra Strength Tylenol, and NSAIDs, such as ibuprofen and naproxen, help for mild symptoms.
- Antidepressants help ease nerve stimulation, which can help nighttime symptoms. Examples include some of the older drugs, such as amitriptyline, nortriptyline, and Tofranil (imipramine), and a newer drug, Cymbalta (duloxetine). Take these at night because they may cause drowsiness and dizziness.
- Antiseizure medications such Neurontin (gabapentin), Topamax (topiramate), Tegretol (carbamazepine), and Lyrica (pregabalin) also quiet nerves. Take these at night also.
- Lidocaine patches contain the anesthetic lidocaine to numb the painful areas.
- A transcutaneous electric nerve stimulation unit is for pain difficult to control by other methods. Electrodes are placed on the skin over painful areas, and a gentle electric current is delivered to mask the neuropathic pain.
- Research is currently underway to test the effects of injecting Botox into the skin on top of the feet to relieve pain.

The most important aspect of taking care of our feet is to prevent amputations. Regardless of whether we have peripheral neuropathy and/or peripheral arterial disease, diabetes itself puts us at risk for this problem. Of course, if you have either or both of these complications you are even more at risk. Constant high blood glucose levels slow down our ability to fight infection anywhere in the body. It is like our immune system and our white blood cells are trying to get to the site of infection in a sea of molasses. By the time they get there, the infection may be well established. Their distance from the heart and the small size of their blood vessels makes fighting infections in the feet most difficult. Therefore, checking feet nightly for redness, warmth, bruising, blisters, and any break in the skin is important. Use magnifying mirrors to see the underside of your feet and toes and in between your toes, because this is where most of the problems occur. Keep mirrors in the bathroom or whereever you are most likely to use them. This may be near the chair where you sit to watch television. Make sure the area is well lighted. Other preventive measures to avoid foot trauma include the following:

- Always wear well-fitting shoes that allow movement of toes, including shower shoes at the gym. Going barefoot can be dangerous for anyone. Glass and stones can cut or bruise feet. Getting athlete's foot from a communal shower, or sliding on a wet tub or tile surface, can happen to anyone but will have more consequences for those of us with diabetes.
- Always check inside shoes before you put them on to feel for debris, tears, sharp edges, or worn areas that might cause irritation or injury to feet.
- Wear seamless socks with shoes to absorb moisture and prevent friction, which could cause a blister.
- Never use sharp implements to treat a callus. See a podiatrist instead.
- Avoid electric blankets, heating pads, or foot soaking products, because these can cause burns and irritation to sensitive skin.
- Use good moisturizing lotions on your feet and heels to keep the skin from cracking.
- Call your healthcare practitioner if you notice any symptoms of peripheral neuropathy or any area of irritation or a blister or ulcer, or any signs of infection on your feet. You need to be seen immediately or within 24 hours. If that is not possible, go to an urgent care center, especially if you have peripheral neuropathy and/or decreased circulation to your feet.

CHARCOT'S JOINT

When a foot has lost most of its sensation, including pain sensation and the ability to sense the position of the joint, muscles also lose their ability to support the joint properly. With an unstable foot, a sprained ankle; inflammation; dislocation; and, eventually, deformity may follow. This neuropathic joint disease, called *Charcot's joint*, after the doctor who first described it, can be very debilitating. People with peripheral neuropathy are at risk for this complication and need to be on the lookout for any symptoms of inflammation, such as swelling, redness, heat, and a strong pulse as well as decreased sensations of the feet. Notify your healthcare provider so your foot can be immobilized with a cast to prevent the progression of any deformity. After the cast is removed, you will need to wear a brace when walking to protect the joint from further damage.

AUTONOMIC NEUROPATHY

Not as common but even more problematic is the nerve damage done to the autonomic nervous system by uncontrolled hyperglycemia. The autonomic nerves regulate body functions that are not under conscious control, such as digestion, heart rate, blood pressure, and bladder and bowel control. Anyone who has autonomic neuropathy probably also has peripheral neuropathy, because the former takes longer to develop. The list of possible problems is long and includes gastroparesis, or slow stomach emptying; neurogenic bladder, or poor bladder control; constipation or diarrhea, or both; rapid or irregular heartbeat, postural drop in blood pressure; difficulty regulating respirations; hypoglycemia unawareness; erectile dysfunction in men; and female sexual dysfunction in the form of frequent yeast infections, vaginal dryness and irritation, decreased libido, and difficulty achieving orgasm. Any of these problems can certainly disrupt a life already complicated by diabetes.

Gastroparesis occurs in five to twelve percent of people with uncontrolled diabetes. Normally, food is broken down by the stomach in about three hours or less, depending on what is eaten. This slurry then moves to the small intestine, where digestive enzymes from the pancreas and the liver (bile) digest the fat, protein, and carbohydrates and begin the process of absorption of these nutrients, as well as the vitamins and minerals they contain. With gastroparesis, food remains in the stomach much longer and symptoms such as fullness and bloating, abdominal pain, heartburn, erratic blood glucose levels, nausea, and vomiting may occur. Controlling blood sugar levels most of the time should prevent this and other types of neuropathy, but once this complication develops blood glucose levels may rise and fall at unanticipated times, making control difficult. Any medication that delays stomach emptying, such as Symlin or Byetta, may make matters worse. Eating six small meals a day and limiting high-fat and high-fiber foods, which also slow stomach emptying, usually help. Liquid or pureed foods may be needed in severe cases. Medications that cause the stomach to contract, moving food into the small intestine, can be prescribed, as can antinausea and antigas drugs. As a last resort, a feeding tube may be surgically inserted into the small intestine to bypass the stomach altogether. This will ensure an intake of adequate nutrients, vitamins, minerals, and calories to avoid malnutrition and make it easier to stabilize blood sugars.

A *neurogenic bladder* is one that does not respond to fullness and the need to urinate, so the bladder may not get emptied. This retained urine can grow bacteria and cause a bladder infection that can force infected urine up into the kidneys, causing kidney damage from the pressure and infection. The converse is also possible, causing urinary incontinence. A person with either problem can be taught to self-catheterize at regular intervals throughout the day. Medication can be prescribed for an overactive bladder as well as for a urinary tract infection, and sometimes surgery can be done to reposition the bladder in women to help with bladder emptying. Both men and women can be taught to use the Credé method, applying manual pressure over the bladder, to enhance emptying.

Hypoglycemia unawareness was covered in Chapter 5, but its root cause is autonomic nerve damage brought on by consistently high blood sugars. People who experience this complication have no warning that a low blood sugar is occurring. They don't have the sweats, shakes, and rapid heartbeat that signal hypoglycemia. This is truly a medical emergency, because if you don't respond to a very low blood glucose level by eating or drinking something to raise your blood sugar you can go into a coma and may have a seizure and/or develop some brain damage. People who develop hypoglycemia unawareness almost always have had type 1 diabetes for many years. They benefit from using a continuous glucose monitoring system, described in Chapter 5, and should be recommended for pancreatic or islet cell transplantation.

Sudomotor neuropathy consists of nerve damage to sweat glands. This can cause excessive sweating and dry skin, which can lead to skin infections, dehydration, and heat stroke. Conversely, it can also hinder your ability to sweat, causing your internal temperature to rise to dangerous levels, resulting in heat stroke. People who experience either of these complication must work at normalizing their blood sugars most of the time, stay hydrated, minimize working or playing in hot weather, and moisturize and check skin for infection daily. Heat stroke should be treated by emergency medical services personnel, who can start an IV and transport the person to an emergency room.

Postural hypotension can prevent blood vessels from automatically constricting when a person goes from sitting or lying down to a standing position. Without this narrowing of blood vessels to increase blood pressure, blood drains from the head by gravity, and the person faints. Other symptoms of this problem include increased heart rate, dizziness, low blood pressure, nausea, and vomiting. To counteract these symptoms, change positions slowly when sitting up from lying down or when standing from a sitting position, and stay near the bed or chair until you no longer feel like passing out. Some people wear compression stockings that help blood return from the legs into the arterial circulation to increase the blood to the brain, and medications to increase blood pressure are available.

Sexual dysfunction can affect both men and women with either type 1 or type 2 diabetes. Autonomic neuropathy from consistently high blood sugars is only one cause of sexual dysfunction. For men with diabetes, this translates to erectile dysfunction, or the inability to have or sustain an erection, especially if combined with poor circulation to the area. In order to have an erection, a man needs to have nervous system stimulation and a rush of blood to the penis. Other health issues that combine to make erectile dysfunction more likely include *hypercholesterolemia*, which clogs arteries and hypertension from constricted arteries. Prevention involves controlling blood glucose levels, blood pressure, and cholesterol levels. TV ads for Viagra, Cialis, and Levetra help to tell the story; however, the success rate of these medications in men with diabetes is only about fifty to sixty percent, which is less than in men without diabetes. A new oral medication, Staxyn, was approved in 2010.

There are other treatments for erectile dysfunction if oral medication does not work, including injections of medication

What Nurses Know...

Drugs for erectile dysfunction can interact with antihypertensive medication, especially alpha blockers and medication for angina, such as nitrates, to cause a dangerous drop in blood pressure. Your healthcare provider needs a list of all of your medications to check for drug-to-drug interactions.

directly into the blood vessels of the penis. This works in sixty to eighty percent of men with diabetes. Vacuum constricting devices also have a high rate of success. They help to achieve and maintain an erection. There are also pellets that can be placed into the urethra as well as surgically implanted penile implants. It sounds to me like maintaining good glucose, blood pressure, and cholesterol control, which would prevent the problem in the first place, is a lot easier.

Female sexual dysfunction doesn't get much press but is equally devastating to the women who experience this complication. Nerve damage to the vagina causes decreased lubrication; decreased or absence of orgasm; vaginal infection with odorous discharge; and vaginismus, a constriction of the vaginal walls that makes penetration painful or impossible. Many women notice that blood sugars are higher or lower than normal the week before the start of their menstrual cycle. Keeping blood sugar records for a couple of months and noting when your period starts may help your healthcare provider see this relationship and help you adjust your medication or insulin, diet, and exercise during these times to help even out the hormonal influences. After menopause is another time when women need to rethink how they are managing their diabetes. Emotions also greatly affect blood glucose. For more on this topic, see Chapter 8. To minimize the likelihood of vaginal infections, practice good hygiene before and after intercourse. Use a vaginal lubricant or estrogen cream suggested or prescribed by your gynecologist if vaginal dryness is a problem. A gynecologist may also have suggestions to increase your libido.

Both men and women with sexual dysfunction need to have their healthcare practitioner review a complete list of prescriptions, over-the-counter medications, and herbal supplements to see whether any of them contribute to this problem. Some have side effects that do. As with all complications, prevention by controlling blood sugars, blood pressure, and cholesterol levels should be your focus.

From the serious and life-threatening complications to the very disconcerting and annoying ones, high blood sugars can affect every body system. In the following sections I discuss a few of the non–life-threatening but bothersome conditions that may strengthen your resolve to work at glucose control.

Teeth and Gum Problems

People with diabetes are at higher risk for developing mouth infections. Bacteria thrive in moist, dark places like the mouth, especially when they have sugar-laden mucous to feast on. The higher our blood sugar, the sweeter all our secretions are, so besides controlling glucose levels we need to brush our teeth at least twice a day with a fluoride toothpaste that also has a bacteria-killing ingredient. Flossing or using another device to keep food particles from lodging between teeth is important. Dental cleaning and checkups at least every six months permit a dental hygienist and/or a dentist to clean and check teeth for cavities and plaque formation and gums for *gingivitis*, the red, swollen, bleeding gums that can lead to *periodontitis*, an inflammation and infection of the gums, ligaments, bones, and other tissue that hold the teeth in place. If pockets of infection form beneath the gum line, a specialized dentist can do procedures such as tooth scaling and root plaining to get rid of the plaque and infection. Often an antibiotic is needed to treat the infection. Consistently high blood sugars (> 200 mg/dl) can lead to periodontitis, but the reverse is also true: Periodontal disease can worsen blood sugar control. If gum disease is not caught early, it can lead to tooth loss.

High blood sugars can also cause *thrush*, a fungal infection of the mouth, tongue, and gums. It looks like white patches that cannot be brushed away and often hurts when any food or liquid, even water, touches it. There are a few antifungal rinses available that can be swished and swallowed to eradicate this infection. Getting a new toothbrush may also be necessary to prevent reinfection. Another common mouth problem is dry mouth, or

What Nurses Know...

When brushing teeth, use a soft toothbrush to avoid causing trauma to gums that might leave an open area for bacteria to invade. Use small, circular motions to remove food and plaque from the gum line and between teeth. When flossing between teeth, use a sawing motion from the gum line to the end of the tooth to avoid cutting into the gum line. If you wear dentures, rinse them and soak them overnight in a liquid made for that purpose, or use an effervescent tablet in water. Chewing sugar-free gum can help to loosen food trapped between teeth and increase saliva production. It can also help in digestion.

xerostomia. This can cause constant bad breath and needs to be treated because the normal amount of saliva helps to keep teeth and gums healthy and free from infection. *Canker sores* may also be an indication that blood glucose levels are out of control. Again, quit smoking, because this makes dry mouth and any gum disease worse. Control stress, because it can make fighting any infection, including periodontitis, more difficult. Blood sugar control really will help you to keep your teeth and your healthy smile.

Be sure to tell your dentist that you have diabetes, and bring him or her a list of all the prescriptions, over-the-counter medications, and herbal supplements you take so the oral care you receive is appropriate for you. Chronic inflammation from gum disease is also associated with heart disease, blocked arteries and stroke, lung infections, preterm labor, and worsening memory and math skills. And you thought it was all about a winning smile.

Musculoskeletal System

Keeping bones, muscles, joints and ligaments healthy and functional depends on keeping blood sugar under control. There are several conditions in this body system that occur more frequently in people who have diabetes than in those without diabetes.

FROZEN SHOULDER

Frozen shoulder (adhesive capsulitis) is a painful restriction of shoulder movement. The capsule of a shoulder joint includes ligaments that attach the arm to the scapula, or shoulder blade, in the upper back, and the arm to the clavicle or collar bone. The shoulder joint is a ball-in-socket joint, which makes it the most versatile joint in our body. It can rotate three hundred sixty degrees (a full circle); can move arms forward, backward, across the chest, and outward away from the body; and reach the back from above and below. The rotator cuff muscles stabilize this joint. Because of all of these useful, everyday movements it can easily be injured when overly stressed. This happens when we attempt to lift, push, pull, or throw something heavier than we are used to. Constant high glucose levels can cause inflammation of many body parts, including muscles and tendons. When inflammation of the capsule occurs, tendons and ligaments get stiff and swollen, and movement is restricted. When movement causes pain, the natural tendency is to not move that joint. Inflammation in joints that are immobile causes adhesions to form, restricting movement even more. The key to regaining full range of motion of the shoulder joint is to reduce the inflammation with good blood sugar control, NSAIDs such as ibuprofen or naproxen, or cortisone injections, and physical therapy. Early and aggressive treatment is necessary. This is truly a case of "move it or lose it." If a significant amount of scar tissue has formed, arthroscopic surgery may be needed. Manipulation of the joint under anesthesia to break up the adhesions is another option. Physical therapy and daily exercising of the shoulder joint after either procedure are absolutely essential to prevent more scar

What Nurses Know...

The body's way of protecting an injured body part is to form a fibrous band of tissue (adhesions, or scar tissue) to protect the body part from further injury. This happens not just in joints but after any surgery.

tissue and adhesions from forming in response to the irritation from surgery.

The importance of controlling blood sugar cannot be overstated. Those of us with diabetes are four times more likely to experience a frozen shoulder, a partial frozen shoulder, or a rotator cuff injury than people who don't have diabetes, but it can still happen to others. I had a partial frozen shoulder years before I was diagnosed with diabetes. Because I got help early, all I needed was physical therapy and daily exercises, such as wall climbing with that arm and doing deep knee bends while holding onto a doorknob with my back to the door, which was doable since I was only in my late twenties. I still do shoulder stretches most days. See Chapter 3 for examples of helpful exercises.

CARPAL TUNNEL SYNDROME

Median nerve entrapment, or *carpal tunnel syndrome*, is often caused by repetitive motion, such typing or painting, that irritates the tendons around the median nerve at the wrist. This causes swelling, which makes the bony tunnel space narrower and compresses the nerve. Hyperglycemia can also add to this inflammation. Numbness, tingling, or a burning sensation of the palm side of your thumb and the first three fingers, as well as pain, sometimes into the forearm, are all reasons to see your healthcare provider. If you also have peripheral neuropathy of

What Nurses Know...

The best anti-inflammatory drug is cortisone, a steroid. Even when it is injected into a joint, it often raises blood sugar for twenty-four to forty-eight hours, so checking blood sugars more often than usual and limiting carbs during this time is a good idea. NSAIDs are usually good alternatives, depending on the degree of inflammation. Note that Tylenol is not an NSAID. It works on pain and fever, but not inflammation.

the hands, there are tests to differentiate between the two. If the problem is carpal tunnel syndrome, then resting the affected hand and wrist, often by wearing a splint, especially at night, is very important. NSAID pain relievers and/or cortisone injections to relieve the inflammation and reduce the swelling are an important part of the treatment.

If splinting and drugs don't cure the problem, carpal tunnel release surgery, which widens the carpal tunnel, may be necessary. This is an outpatient procedure done under local anesthesia. If you do nothing about this problem, the consequence is more than living with pain: The nerve can be permanently damaged and the thumb muscles can atrophy or wither. And, of course, controlling blood sugar is important to prevent this condition from coming back.

TRIGGER FINGER

Flexor tenosynovitis, also called *trigger finger*, is an irritation and narrowing of the sheath that surrounds the flexor tendon, causing it to catch and release like a trigger. The most common finger affected is the ring finger of either hand, but any finger—or the thumbs, for that matter—can be involved. You'd think it would more likely happen on your dominant hand, but I've had two fingers and the thumb of my left hand, and only the ring finger of my right hand, surgically repaired so far. The cause of such minor annoyances is the same as with all other muscle or tendon inflammation. Blood glucose control matters, but how long a person has had diabetes seems to matter more. People whose work or hobbies require repeated gripping actions, such as knitting or crocheting, whether or not they have diabetes, are more susceptible. The first time it happened to me was caused by tightly gripping the steering wheel for a tense forty-minute commute to work on mostly interstate highways. It is more common in women and in anyone with diabetes.

Nonsurgical interventions can include splinting the finger(s) or thumb, especially while sleeping, to prevent you from curling your fingers into a ball. You can also do this by placing your hand, palm down and fingers straight, under your pillow. Gentle finger massage from the palm down the affected finger(s) or thumb and warm soaks may give temporary relief. The use of NSAIDs and

What Nurses Know...

NAIDs like ibuprofen (Advil, Motrin, etc.) or naproxen (Aleve and others) must be taken with or after food, even crackers; otherwise, they may irritate the stomach lining and, over time, cause a stomach ulcer to form. All of these meds work like aspirin in that they prevent platelets from sticking together and forming a clot. However, if you are also taking other drugs that prevent clotting, such as Coumadin or Plavix, your body's ability to clot when needed may be compromised, leading to excessive bruising (bleeding under the skin) or, potentially, hemorrhaging.

cortisone injections may be useful to relieve the inflammation and swelling.

For a more permanent solution to a trigger finger, an orthopedic hand surgeon may perform a percutaneous (performed through the skin) release of the affected tendon or a surgical release. Both are outpatient procedures done under local anesthesia. For a good picture of a trigger finger check out the Mayo Clinic's Web site at www.mayoclinic.com/health/trigger-finger/ds00155/dsection=risk-factors, or the American Academy of Orthopedic Surgeons site at http://orthoinfo.aaos.org/topic.cfm?topic=a00024. After the bulky dressing and stitches are removed, you will need to gently message the palm and finger(s) or thumb and stretch them to get full extension. Compare the surgical hand with your other hand to see how far back the fingers should go. Keep working on the operated fingers or thumb several times a day until they look like the ones on the other hand. This can take several weeks to months.

Skin Problems

Dry skin is common for people with diabetes, and applications of a good emollient, such as Vaseline Intensive Care, Gold Bond, or

What Nurses Know . . .

Any open wound, even just a crack, cut, or abrasion, should be checked often for signs of infection. Any redness, puffiness, warmth, or oozing should be seen by a healthcare practitioner immediately. Even a mild infection can easily get out of hand when you have diabetes. An infection also raises blood sugar, and increased glucose levels make infections worse.

Aveeno lotion daily is very important, especially on the heels and feet to prevent cracking that can open up the skin for bacteria to enter. Never put lotion in between toes, because this provides a good medium for fungus to grow. With any break in the skin, an antibiotic cream should be applied and the wound covered with a water-resistant adhesive bandage. Once it starts to close, leave it open to air at least at night if it needs to be protected, depending on its location, during the day.

DIABETIC DERMOPATHY

This condition consists of roundish, slightly indented brown or purplish patches, usually over the shin bones. It may occur after many years with diabetes. It does not hurt and usually does not itch. It may fade with improved blood sugar control. A low dose of chelated zinc tablets taken daily for several weeks, especially if combined with near-normal glucose levels, may help. Talk it over with your healthcare practitioner.

ACANTHOSIS NIGRICANS

This skin problem results in the darkening and thickening of skin, especially in creases. The skin may be slightly raised. It is more common in very overweight individuals, often indicates insulin resistance, and usually precedes the diagnosis of type 2 diabetes. Blood sugar control and weight loss may improve this condition.

NECROBIOSIS LIPOIDICA

This skin disease occurs in the lower legs and often indicates reduced blood supply to the skin. The skin becomes thinned and reddened. Trauma to the area can cause ulceration. It can be itchy and painful. Good blood sugar control usually prevents it, and ulcers need to be treated to prevent infections.

FUNGAL INFECTIONS

Because sustained high blood glucose levels put your immune system in sleep mode, it is easy to see why people who don't control blood sugars are susceptible to infections. Fungi and bacteria need to be fed to grow, and glucose in bodily secretions, blood, sweat, and on the skin is a perfect food. They also like warm, dark, moist areas. Fungi grow well between the toes as athlete's foot; in the groin area as jock itch; in the vagina as a yeast infection; and in the mouth as thrush; as well as in the armpits, under the foreskin, and under the breasts. *Ringworm* is a ring-shaped itchy patch caused by a fungus (no worm involved). It can also grow under nails and around nail beds. Antifungal creams and/or oral antifungal medication may be needed to treat these infections. Blood sugar control is also needed.

BACTERIAL INFECTIONS

If that last paragraph didn't gross you out enough, let me list the various bacterial infections that can plague those who are not motivated to live a healthy lifestyle and work at controlling blood sugars. Bacteria that are allowed to multiply on and under the skin can cause boils and carbuncles (deeper and larger than boils), a stye (infection of the glands of the eyelids), folliculites (infection of the hair follicles), and infections around toenails and fingernails. Staph skin infections need to be treated with oral antibiotics, good hygiene, and blood glucose control.

WOUND CARE

When there is a break in the skin anywhere, those of us with diabetes need to be worried. A minor wound can be cleansed with soap and water and an over-the-counter antibiotic ointment and covered with a Band-Aid large enough to cover and pad the area. Gauze and paper or surgical tape can also be used.

If a wound is extensive and/or deep, seeing a healthcare provider or going to an urgent care center is a must. Any infected wound can become a major wound. If your diabetes is not treated with insulin, you may be put on insulin until the wound is on its way to being healed and the infection is gone. If you usually inject or pump insulin, you will probably need to take a higher dose. You will also need to take an antibiotic by mouth, injection, or IV,

What Nurses Know . . .

When you get a cut, change the dressing at least once a day. Wash the area with soap and water, and dry carefully. Observe the wound itself for healing. It should go from red or bleeding to oozing pink and then clear fluid. Then you should notice the formation of a scab. When a scab starts to form, keep it clean and expose it to air unless it needs to be padded to protect it from injury during the day. Look for signs of infection, such as the area around the wound getting red, swollen, hot, or drainage that is green or bright yellow. It may also have an odor, and your blood sugars might be higher. If you notice any of these signs, see your healthcare practitioner as soon as possible.

which may necessitate hospitalization. Special dressings may be needed and, depending on the wound's location, a cast, special shoes, bed rest, or a special mattress to keep the pressure off the wound or ulcer may be ordered. This is nothing to fool around with.

If, despite all your efforts, you develop a complication or two, remember that there are lots of treatments, as listed in this chapter, and more on the horizon. Also know that what you are experiencing would have happened sooner and been worse if you had not worked so hard at controlling your glucose levels. Seek help early and work with your healthcare team to stay on top of whatever you are confronting. Diabetes management is not an exact science. Human error, whether through carelessness or willful inattention, accounts for most of the ups and downs of blood sugars. However, as long as we continue to work on being as healthy as we can, we can feel good about ourselves no matter what the numbers on the glucose meter are. Look at the meter numbers as a learning experience. If there is no apparent reason for a high reading, record it and move on. Dwelling on it will take away from the joy of living, as will excessive worry about complication. Keeping a log of what, when, and how much you eat; what, when, and how much you exercise; and what your blood sugar levels are will be important in putting the pieces of the puzzle together so you can understand how they relate. Successful people of any age, in any walk of life, facing any challenge, medical or otherwise, all have one thing in common: They take the cards they were dealt and play them to the best of their ability. Win, lose, or draw, they meet my definition of success.

This may have been a hard chapter for you to read. It was a hard chapter for me to write. If you skipped through and read only those areas about which you had questions, you know where to find more answers. Read more when you have questions or need more information. We are all human and thus certainly not perfect. Doing the best you can under the circumstances is all you can ask of yourself. To quote Helen Keller, "When one door closes, another opens; but often we look so long at the closed door that we do not see the one which has opened for us."

Diabetes and Pregnancy

I have had diabetes since I was ten years old and would like to have a baby. Can I? Is it safe for me and the baby?   DONNA

My last baby was over ten pounds, and I needed a [cesarean] section. My doctor told me I had gestational diabetes. Can I prevent this from happening this time?   JUNE

If you are planning a pregnancy and have diabetes, like Donna, or have had gestational diabetes mellitus (GDM) with your last pregnancy, like June, the information in this chapter may be of particular interest to you.

Diabetes and Pregnancy

PREGESTATIONAL DIABETES

Many women often wonder about the effects of pregnancy on their body, but women with preexisting diabetes have good reason to be concerned.

Type 1 Diabetes   Years ago, women with type 1 diabetes diagnosed as children were discouraged from getting pregnant. Prior
to the development of insulin in 1922, children with diabetes did
not live long enough to procreate. Anyone who remembers seeing the 1989 film *Steel Magnolias* is aware that pregnancy can
cause damage to glucose-sensitive organs in women with type
1 diabetes. In the film, Julia Roberts plays a woman with type 1
childhood-onset diabetes. She is warned not to attempt pregnancy by her physician and her mother. She does so anyway, has
a difficult time with the pregnancy and delivery, and ends up
dying of renal failure a year later. Even though many advances
have been made in the care of pregnant women in general, and
those with diabetes in particular, many parents of young diabetic women may still consider pregnancy a death sentence for
their daughters. More sophisticated glucose meters, rapid-acting
insulin, insulin pumps, and research have greatly impacted the
safety of pregnancy for women with diabetes. More women with
long-standing disease have fewer complications today due to better glycemic control before pregnancy that decreases potential
complications.

Pregnancy for anyone is considered a complex metabolic state
that causes dramatic shifts in glucose, fat, and protein utiliza-
tion. During the first trimester, the body is insulin sensitive and
burns more fat for energy than usual, thus decreasing insulin
demands. Many women are also nauseated, and normal weight
gain is typically less than four pounds during this time. Some
women actually lose weight because of nausea and vomiting. As
the placenta becomes fully functional during the second trimester, it produces increasing amount of hormones (human placental
growth hormone, human placental lactogen, and progesterose)
that cause insulin resistance. By the third trimester, the pancreas
must produce up to three times the amount of insulin for the
body to remain normoglycemic. In addition, the basal metabolic
rate increases tremendously, and both the woman's demands for
glucose and those of her fetus are considerable. Normally, weight
gain during the second and third trimesters equals up to one

pound per week, with a total weight gain of twenty-five to thirty-five pounds expected. During a normal pregnancy, women have a lower fasting glucose level and produce more insulin than when they are not pregnant because of the increase in glucose uptake by the fetus and the placenta as well as by the cells of their own body. With a normal pancreas, the added insulin needs are fulfilled automatically. When an actual diabetic state is added to the normal changes in pregnancy, glycemic control is further challenged. The consequences of not controlling blood sugars for a pregnant woman can include a worsening of any preexisting long-term complications, such as retinopathy, nephropathy, neuropathy, hypertension, and cardiovascular disease. Even without preexisting diabetic complications, women with type 1 diabetes are at increased risked for pregnancy-induced hypertension, miscarriage, and diabetic ketoacidosis, as well as the beginning of chronic long-term complications, if glycemic control is not achieved. Therefore, preconception care for women with diabetes focuses on achieving blood sugar control. This is important to prevent miscarriages and birth defects. Maternal hyperglycemia can cause damage to the embryo in the first few weeks of gestation, when organ formation is taking place. This may be occurring before a women even knows she is pregnant. With uncontrolled glucose levels later on in pregnancy, the fetus grows larger than normal (*macrosomia*), making vaginal birth difficult or impossible. This increases the likelihood of difficulty delivering the shoulders, a fractured clavicle, or the need for a cesarean delivery. Hyperglycemia also increases the incidence of stillbirths. The infant of a diabetic mother with uncontrolled blood sugars is at risk for jaundice, respiratory distress syndrome (especially if the baby is large), and prematurity even if the baby is large. Macrosomic babies usually have more fat cells than normal and are at risk for obesity and type 2 diabetes during their lifetimes.

Type 2 Diabetes Women with pregestational type 2 diabetes are often overweight and may have hypertension. It is as important for these women to prepare for pregnancy as it is for women with type 1 diabetes. A study conducted by T. D. Clausen and others that compared women with type 2 diabetes with women with type 1 diabetes and those without diabetes concluded that fetal and newborn mortality increased by four to nine times, and major birth defects were more than doubled, in women with type 2 diabetes. Type 2 diabetes is a lot more than just "a touch of sugar." The women in this study were older, overweight, had more children, were often non-White, with a shorter duration of time since diagnosis, and had A1cs during pregnancy that were lower than women with type 1 diabetes. This seems to be counterintuitive. However, most clients with type 1 diabetes were in better glycemic control before pregnancy, planned the pregnancy, sought prenatal care earlier, were of normal weight, and were younger, with fewer pregnancies than women with type 2 diabetes in this study. Many of the women with type 2 diabetes had metabolic syndrome and were insulin resistant prior to pregnancy. This study points out the importance to women with type 2 diabetes of preparing the body for pregnancy by losing weight; controlling blood pressure; and controlling blood sugars, often with insulin, because most oral agents can cause birth defects in the first trimester. Glyburide, a sulfonylurea, has been given to women after twenty-four weeks of gestation and was shown not to cross the placenta or cause any fetal problems. This might be a good choice for treatment of GDM, which develops about this time. Metformin (Glucophage) can be used in the first trimester for women with polycystic ovarian syndrome (PCOS) to reverse infertility and prevent an early miscarriage; however, there is an increased risk of developing pregnancy-induced hypertension and, because this drug does cross the placenta, there is an increased risk of fetal abnormalities.

GESTATIONAL DIABETES MELLITUS

GDM is diagnosed only during the latter half of pregnancy. Blood sugars usually return to normal after delivery of the placenta. The placental hormones mentioned earlier cause increasing insulin resistance as the pregnancy progresses and may outpace the pancreas's ability to increase insulin production in some women. The screening tool for GDM given to pregnant women between twenty-four and twenty-eight weeks consists of a glucose challenge test. A 50-g Glucola solution is administered orally, and a serum glucose is obtained one hour later. A blood sugar greater than 130 mg/dl will identify around ninety percent of women who have gestational diabetes. This subset of women should then receive a three-hour, 100-g oral glucose tolerance test (OGTT). See below for criteria for a positive three-hour OGTT.

THREE-HOUR OGTT DIAGNOSTIC CRITERIA FOR GDM

Fasting ≥ 95 mg/dl
1 hour ≥ 180 mg/dl
2 hours ≥ 155 mg/dl
3 hours ≥ 140 mg/dl

Meeting or exceeding any two values is regarded as a positive test and is diagnostic of GDM. If only one value is met or exceeded, a repeat three-hour OGTT is scheduled one month later.

Reprinted with permission from Diabetes Care, Vol. 33, 2010; S11-S61. © 2010 American Diabetes Association.

The American Diabetes Association (2010) recommends testing pregnant women at very high risk for GDM as soon as the pregnancy is confirmed using an A1c test. The criteria for very high risk include the following:

- Severe obesity
- Prior history of GDM
- Delivery of a large-for-gestational-age baby
- Presence of glucose in the urine
- Diagnosis of PCOS
- Strong family history of type 2 diabetes

If the A1c is 6.5 or greater, type 2 diabetes is diagnosed. If it is not, then the screening test described earlier is done at twenty-

What Nurses Know...

A one-hour glucose challenge test can be done at any time of day without fasting or any other preparation. When a three-hour OGTT is scheduled, you must have fasted for at least eight hours overnight after three days of carbohydrate loading consisting of a daily intake of about 200 g of carbohydrates. Choose from fruits (15 g); breads (15 g); cereal (15–30 g); rice (15 g); pasta (15 g); milk or yogurt (12–20g); and starchy vegetables (15 g) such as potatoes, beans, or corn.

four to twenty-eight weeks of gestation along with all other women who are not in the low-risk category. Low-risk pregnant women include those with the following characteristics:

1. Younger than 25 years
2. Normal weight prior to pregnancy
3. No known diabetes in first-degree relatives (parents, siblings)
4. No history of poor pregnancy outcomes
5. No history of abnormal glucose tolerance
6. No ancestry from a high-risk population (African Americans; Asian Americans; Native American Indians; Mexican American; and Pacific Islanders, such as Hawaiians and Filipinos)

GDM represents most of all pregnancies complicated by diabetes. With the obesity rates of women in their childbearing years (ages fifteen through forty-four) increasing, the rate of GDM likely will increase in the near future. This diagnosis increases the risk for these women of being diagnosed with type 2 diabetes, often within five to ten years of the pregnancy. Three abnormalities make glucose regulation during pregnancy more difficult than normal for women diagnosed with GDM: (1) insulin resistance, which is common in the third trimester for all women; (2) glucose metabolism, which in women with GDM is further hampered by impaired insulin secretion; and (3) increased liver glucose production. Their insulin resistance is greater than in normal pregnancies during the third trimester, thus compounding the problem, resulting in hyperglycemia. The good news about GDM is that it goes away once you deliver the placenta and its anti-insulin hormones. You will need to continue to have your blood sugars checked while you are in the hospital to make sure you don't really have type 2 diabetes, and they will be checked again at your postpartum visit. Once a year you may be asked to have another OGTT or tested with an A1c to diagnose type 2 diabetes. Weight loss and exercise are your best defense against developing diabetes. You will be followed closely and early with each pregnancy for a return of GDM. If you remain as fit and trim as possible, you may be able to avoid GDM in the future.

Motivation in Pregnant Women With Diabetes

The preceding information should motivate women with diabetes to work at controlling blood sugars before and during pregnancy. Following your A1c levels every three months will help you evaluate the success of your efforts and indicate when attempting pregnancy is optimal. If you do not see a healthcare professional on a regular basis, you are more likely to become pregnant without the benefit of good glycemic control and may well develop some of the complications discussed earlier. When most women plan a pregnancy, they are excited and eager to have a healthy, uncomplicated pregnancy and birth. They usually are motivated to eat a healthy diet, get some exercise, and follow any advice given. This may be the best time for you to pay attention to advice

NORMAL GLUCOSE LEVELS AND A1CS DURING THE SECOND AND THIRD TRIMESTER

Group	Average glucose	Fasting, premeal, bedtime	One hour after meals	A1c
Normal nonpregnant	97–125	70–99	123–137	5.0–5.9
Normal pregnancy	77.1–88.7	63.6–75	102.4–114.4	5.0
Goals during 2nd & 3rd trimesters with preexisting diabetes	<110	60–99	100–129	<6.2

about achieving good glycemic control. Blood sugar ranges during pregnancy are the same for diabetic and nondiabetic women alike, a point that should make you feel normal perhaps for the first time since your diagnosis. These ranges shown in the chart above are about twenty percent lower than for people who are not pregnant.

These levels are, however, easy to achieve in nondiabetic women because their needed increase in insulin is automatic. Those who cannot overcome the pregnancy-induced insulin resistance by producing more and more insulin as the pregnancy progresses develop GDM. Because GDM increases the risk for complications during pregnancy and the risk of a large baby complicating delivery, you should also be acutely interested in learning how to control blood sugars. The following list of topics should be covered by your healthcare practitioner. Be aware that these are areas of concern for general diabetic care as well as good glycemic control during pregnancy and should be continued after pregnancy.

1. Glucose monitoring should be done at least before meals and at bedtime. Women with type 2 diabetes and GDM should periodically test two hours after a meal. Following your two-hour postprandial blood glucose levels will indicate whether

appropriate steps are being taken to control glucose spikes, which are most strongly correlated with fetal macrosomia.

2. A registered dietitian may be needed to review your current eating habits and make appropriate recommendations for change as needed. Diets that do not accommodate your likes and dislikes or your financial situation are a waste of time and effort. Speak up so your meal plan will meet the nutritional requirements of pregnancy and be appropriate for you. Decreasing carbohydrates to forty-five percent of the total calories you consume may be necessary to blunt postprandial blood sugars if you have type 2 diabetes or GDM. If you are overweight, it might be necessary to decrease not only carbohydrate intake but also the total amount of calories. An average nonpregnant American woman who is not overweight has a caloric intake of 2,400 kcal per day. Pregnant women need to increase this amount by roughly three hundred forty calories during the second trimester to account for the increase in maternal tissue (breast, uterus, blood supply) and the placenta and fetus.

What Nurses Know . . .

·Women at various stages should consume the following nutrients per day.

Nutrients	Adult woman	2nd trimester	3rd trimester	Breastfeeding
Calories	2,400	2,740	2,852	2,700
Protein	100–120 g	130–170 g	130–170 g	130–170 g
Carbs	130 g	175 g	175 g	210 g
Total fiber	25 g	28 g	28 g	29 g
Folate	400 mcg	600 mcg	600 mcg	500 mcg
Iron	8 mg	27 mg	27 mg	9 mg

During the third trimester calories should increase by four hundred fifty-two calories per day to provide for the growth of the fetus. No extra calories are needed during the first trimester. With breastfeeding, roughly three hundred more calories over a nonpregnant intake are needed to produce breast milk with the amount of fat, protein, nutrients and increased fluid volume needed by the baby.

These numbers of calories might be a drastic reduction for you if you have type 2 diabetes or GDM. However, this caloric amount should achieve a pregnancy weight gain of around fifteen pounds for those of you who are overweight, resulting in a normal size baby (seven to eight pounds) and an actual weight loss for you postpartum.

A diet low in fat, moderate in animal protein, and high in whole grains and fiber with five to nine servings of fresh fruit and vegetables and four servings of low-fat dairy should meet the needs of pregnancy.

3. Moderate exercise is recommended for all pregnant women. It is particularly important to help maintain glycemic control if you have diabetes. The concern for anyone who is pregnant

What Nurses Know...

Total weight gain during pregnancy for anyone not overweight with only one fetus should be between twenty-five and thirty-five pounds. The increased folic acid and very high iron requirements during pregnancy may need to be supplemented with the addition of prenatal vitamins in the second and third trimesters, even with a very nutritious diet.

is to avoid exceeding a heart rate of one hundred fifty beats per minute. Prevention of dehydration and heat exhaustion is important, because these conditions affect the baby as well. Low-impact aerobic, weight-bearing exercise three times per week should greatly enhance your feeling of well-being. If you are taking insulin you should exercise after eating or test your blood sugar before exercising and eat something if it is less than 150 mg/dl to prevent hypoglycemia during and after exercise.

4. Insulin does not cross the placenta and is the drug of choice for women with either type 1 or type 2 diabetes during pregnancy. If you have type 2 diabetes and are taking pills to control your diabetes, you may be switched to insulin prior to pregnancy. If you are taking antihypertensives, especially ACE (angiotensin-converting enzyme) inhibitors or ARBs (angiotensin receptor blockers), other medication will be substituted because these drugs may cause birth defects. The literature supports use of older antihypertensives, such as methyldopa (Aldomet), hydralazine (Apresoline), and nifedipine (Procardia), during pregnancy. If you have been diagnosed with GDM you may be able to control blood sugars with diet and exercise and/or may need medication such as glyburide after twenty-four weeks, or insulin.

5. Breastfeeding, once you deliver, is generally recommended even after a cesarean delivery because it helps to stabilize blood sugars. If you are on insulin, your requirements may be twenty-five percent lower than before pregnancy. Insulin does appear in breast milk, but the infant's gastric juices destroy it so the baby does not absorb any of it. Some of you with type 2 diabetes may not need any medication at all while breastfeeding as long as you continue the healthy eating and exercise habits you developed during pregnancy. Oral dia-betic medication should not be taken while breastfeeding, so if you need medication it will have to be insulin. Anyone who breastfeeds for one year reduces her risk of developing type 2 diabetes by fourteen percent. Breastfeeding also helps your

infant by protecting him or her from obesity and early development of type 1 diabetes. Breastfeed for as long as you can. It is the healthiest thing you can do for you and your baby. Most pediatricians prefer that infants drink either breast milk or formula for the first twelve month of life, so breastfeeding is also very economical.

You need to express your concerns to your healthcare provider about planning for pregnancy; how pregnancy may affect diabetes control, and vice versa; and what you can anticipate during labor, delivery, and the postpartum period. Pregnancy, although high risk, is safe for women who have diabetes, especially if blood glucose levels are fairly well controlled (A1c of 7%) prior to and during the pregnancy and advice from your healthcare team is followed.

One last motivating point if you are pregnant and have diabetes or GDM is the fact that you can be a positive role model for your children and your whole family by serving and eating a healthy diet and by increasing physical activity.

GENETIC IMPLICATIONS OF DIABETES

In the beginning of this book I discussed my guilt for bringing this disease into my family and adding to the list of familial diseases in my children's medical history. After some research, I discovered that their risk of contracting type 1 diabetes was very small. Diabetes is caused by genetic factors and environmental factors. Most individuals with type 1 diabetes have inherited risk factors from both parents. It also is more prevalent in the White race. In order for this genetic factor to become manifest, there must be an environmental trigger. Research studies have isolated cold weather and certain viruses as possible triggers. Breastfeeding infants and feeding solids only after six months of age seems to be protective. Because type 1 diabetes is an autoimmune disease, those who may get type 1 diabetes usually have autoantibodies in their blood. Siblings of people with type 1 diabetes could be tested for these autoantibodies to pancreatic beta cells. Type 2 diabetes has a much stronger genetic component. A family history of type 2 diabetes is a very strong risk factor for getting the disease; however, other components, such as obesity; a high-fat, low-fiber diet; and a sedentary lifestyle may make the difference between one family member who develops the disease and another who does not. According to D. Dabelea and others (2005), women who are diagnosed with GDM more often than not were infants of a mother with GDM. The American Diabetes Association lists on their Web site the following genetic statistics. A child of a person with the listed characteristics has the following chance of developing the same type of diabetes:

1. Male with type 1 → child 1 in 17
2. Female with type 1 birthing child before age 25 → child 1 in 25
3. Female with type 1 birthing child after age 25 → child 1 in 100
4. Both parents have type 1 diabetes → child between 1 in 10 to 1 in 4
5. Male or female with type 2 diagnosed before age 50 → child 1 in 7
6. Type 2 diagnosed after age 50 → child 1 in 13
7. Mother has type 2 → child at increased risk
8. Both parents with type 2 → child 1 in 2

The prevalence of type 2 diabetes in some families is clearly genetic but also has a learned behavior component. Families often teach children by example, including behavior such as poor food choices as well as avoidance of physical activity. It is my hope that, by reading this chapter and this book, those of you who are parents are convinced you can turn this around for your children's sake as well as to control your own diabetes. Be motivated and empowered to do so.

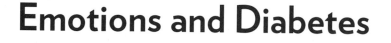

Emotions and Diabetes

Every time I get upset my blood sugar goes high. This makes me angry, and I feel out of control. I have a stressful job and I just can't quit to take care of my diabetes. What can I do to keep my emotions and my blood sugars normal?   SANDY

In the Introduction, I wrote about the stages of grief that usually occur when a diagnosis of diabetes (or any other illness) is given and how I experienced them. Even though emotional responses are necessary to get to acceptance of a diagnosis so you can move forward, they still affect blood sugar, as Sandy stated. Emotions such as depression, anger and frustration, stress, fear and anxiety, and a host of others can increase blood sugar by causing the release of stress hormones such as adrenalin, as stated in Chapter 5. Emotions also may cause us to lose focus on what we are eating, decrease physical activity, omit testing blood glucose levels, and forget to take medication. As human beings we can't avoid these negative feelings. We need to learn how to deal with them in a productive way that should result in a feeling of empowerment and control. Even positive emotions such as joy, happiness, gratitude, hope, and love can have an effect on blood glucose levels. Testing blood sugars more often during times of intense emotion may help to convince us that moderating these emotions may also help to control blood glucose levels.

Negative Emotions

Negative emotions are often counterproductive. They cause us to lose sight of what we are trying to accomplish and may derail our efforts to control blood sugars. They also may cause damage to the cardiovascular system, so it is worth taking a look at each one, the symptoms, and possible treatments to help you regain control of your life as soon as possible.

DEPRESSION

Which comes first: Are you depressed because you have diabetes, or did depression play a role in causing this disease? Does it really matter? Having a diagnosis like diabetes puts you at higher risk for depression. If you think you might be depressed, getting help is what matters. Depression can cause you to make less effort to control blood sugar. You may eat inappropriately; eat too much, or not enough; sleep too much, or be unable to get sufficient rest; forget to monitor your blood glucose level; or become more physically inactive. You may have trouble concentrating; lose the ability to enjoy life; or obsess about some picky thing, experience anxiety or guilt, or be excessively nervous and agitated. Physical aches and pains, including headaches as well as nausea and vomiting can also be part of the symptoms of depression. You may even feel like the situation is so hopeless that you contemplate suicide. There are enough ads on TV for antidepressant medications that you or your family members may easily recognize most symptoms of depression.

Sometimes depression may manifest itself differently, however. The intense anger I felt when my mother died surprised me and had its root in depression. It caused me to inappropriately lose my temper and say and do things that probably made those at work and at home wonder about my sanity. But nobody, including me, thought I was depressed. I started seeing a psychologist because I knew I needed to do *something.* She diagnosed a situational depression. After a few weeks on medication, I felt better and was able to get control of my blood sugars. Afterward, I read through my log book and realized that I had been monitoring blood sugars, which were usually high, and giving myself, insulin, but I had no recollection of doing so. All I remembered was that I was mad a lot and could not seem to control my anger.

According to the National Institutes of Health, more than 20 million adults in the United States suffer from depression. Depression affects twice as many women as men, and most people with depression try to ignore it and do not seek help. They may not recognize the symptoms they are experiencing as depression, they may fear social stigma from needing psychiatric help, or the symptoms may be so debilitating that they cannot reach out for help.

What Nurses Know...

If you have ever experienced any form of depression, such as seasonal affective disorder; postpartum depression; or depression after a life-changing event, like a death in the family; or if you have a family history of depression, you are at higher risk. Symptoms of depression usually do not go away on their own. Depression also weakens the immune system, increasing vulnerability to physical illnesses.

If you think you are experiencing depression, or someone close to you suggests that you might be, the good news is that it is very treatable. Seeking help early will increase the likelihood that your depression will not lead to a more debilitating situation. Here are some suggestions for dealing with depression:

- Psychotherapy or therapeutic talk time with a mental health professional is a great place to start if your depression is mild and not overwhelming. A therapist can help you examine any problems or difficulties that may have led to depression. Sometimes the cause may not be what you think it is. By talking about your situation you are using your therapist as a sounding board. By verbalizing our emotions to someone else, we have to attach words to these thoughts and make them more specific and real. Listening to our own descriptions of these feelings may help us understand them better. When the therapist listens to you, he or she can help you find better ways of coping and develop new thought patterns and behavior toward any life situation.

- Cognitive behavioral therapy is a short-term (ten to twenty sessions) therapy with a mental health professional that is very useful for mild depression. The therapist helps the depressed person to identify and change negative self-talk to more realistic and positive self-talk. The more negative we are about our skills and abilities, the more hopeless and depressed we are about any situation we face and the more we blame ourselves for the mess we perceive we are in. By helping us to think more positively and realistically about ourselves and how we interact with our world, the therapist can redirect negative assumptions and work with us to develop a more hopeful and optimistic view of life. To find a therapist, look in the Resources section in the back of this book under "American Psychological Association."

- Medication can help with depression by increasing the levels of neurotransmitters in the brain. These neurotransmitters include serotonin, norepinephrine, and dopamine, which are needed for the brain to function optimally. They also control mood and may be prescribed in addition to or in place of psychotherapy. This is particularly true if you are suffering from a major depression, have had suicidal thoughts, or if you are having trouble simply living your daily life.

Because psychotherapy takes a number of weeks and months, you can do several things to help ensure this therapy will work. Scale back some of your responsibilities. If you had a physical ailment, you would not take on added responsibilities and would probably relinquish some of what you are currently doing until you felt better. If you have an emotional ailment, you should treat it similarly. Break tasks up into small parts so you can feel you have accomplished something before moving on to the next part. Minimize the time you spend alone, even if you just sit there with family and friends and don't participate in the conversation. Being alone may make you ruminate about perceived

What Nurses Know...

Do not discontinue any medication without your medical provider's supervision. Abruptly stopping medication can cause symptoms of withdrawal, which can lead to a worsening of depression. Antidepressants are typically taken for four to six months. In some cases, however, clients and their doctors may decide that antidepressants are needed for a longer period of time. While on any antidepressant, avoid drinking alcoholic beverages. The interaction can intensify the sedative effects of some antidepressants. Chronic alcohol use can increase the levels of some antidepressants in your blood while decreasing the levels of others.

Classification	Medication	Function	Side Effects
Selective serotonin reuptake inhibitors (SSRIs)	Celexa (citalopram) Lexapro (escitalopram) Prozac (fluoxetine) Paxil (paroxetine) Zoloft (sertraline)	Slows the removal of serotonin in the brain, making more of it available for brain function, mood control	Dry mouth, nausea, nervousness, insomnia, headache, and sexual problems
Serotonin and norepinephrine reuptake inhibitors (SNRIs)	Cymbalta (duloxetine) Effexor (venlafaxine) Pristiq (desvenlafaxine)	Slows the removal of serotonin and norepinephrine in the brain	Nausea, loss of appetite, anxiety, nervousness, headache, insomnia, and tiredness
Dopamine and norepinephrine reuptake inhibitors	Wellbutrin (bupropion)	Slows the removal of dopamine and norepinephrine	Agitation, insomnia, headache, and nausea
Atypical antipsychotics (may be added to other antidepressants)	Abilify (aripiprazole) Desyrel (trazodone) Risperdal (risperidone) Seroquel (quetiapine) Serzone (nefazodone) Zyprexa (olanzapine)	Slows the removal of serotonin, dopamine, and norepinephrine in the brain	Nausea, fatigue, weight gain, dry mouth, sleepiness, nervousness, and blurred vision
Tricyclics	Elavil (amitriptyline) Norpramin (desipramine) Pamelor (nortriptyline) Remeron (mirtazapine) Tofranil (imipramine)	Slows the removal of serotonin and norepinephrine in the brain, may also interact with other chemicals throughout the body	Drowsiness, dry mouth, blurred vision, constipation, difficulty urinating, worsening of glaucoma, impaired thinking, and tiredness

failures, increase a sense of guilt, and make you more depressed. Participate in activities that in the past you have enjoyed, such as mild exercise or going to a movie, a ball game, a church service, or some other social event. Postpone making any life decisions such as changing jobs, or getting married or divorced, until your depression has lifted. Do not expect to *snap out* of your depression. Confide in a family member or friend who can help you troubleshoot any interference from others who do not understand your situation. Continue to see your therapist, and stay on your medication, if needed, even if you do not see an immediate gain. It takes time to undo and replace negative thinking with more positive feelings.

The Food and Drug Administration has ordered makers of all antidepressant medications to include a "black box warning" (the most serious warning level) on their products' labeling. It includes information about increased risks of suicidal thinking and behavior in children, adolescents, and young adults (ages eighteen to twenty-four) during initial treatment (generally the first one to two months). The table above includes current medications for depression (with the generic name in parentheses) with their classifications as well as the function and side effects of each classification. Many people do not experience any side effects and those who do often experience fewer and milder symptoms as time goes on.

ANGER AND FRUSTRATION

If you respond to negative events in your life with anger and/or frustration, you need to find and work on new and less problematic means of dealing with them. If you think "Why me?" or "This isn't fair," you are correct. There is nothing fair about diabetes. When I was first diagnosed with diabetes I had several unexplained (at least to me at the time) high blood sugars that made me want to throw my glucose meter against the wall. Because this first meter cost me $300 out of pocket, I was able to restrain myself. Instead, I yelled and talked nasty to myself and took my frustrations out on things I could throw that would not break.

Then I worked on why this happened, but often I could not figure it out, which increased my frustration. After a year or so of
dealing with this I came to the conclusion that *why* did not matter as much as fixing the high blood sugar did. Beating yourself
up about high blood sugars is counterproductive. Getting a high
blood sugar back to normal should be your focus, unless the reason for the high is easily and readily discovered.

One of the most frustrating things about having diabetes is its
24/7 demands. Unlike the commitment to raising children, who
eventually grow up, diabetes never goes away. If you've seen the
TV commercials for Onglyza, you may relate to the person who
exercises and tries to eat right but continues to have high blood
sugars. The frustration and anger felt when you really are trying
to do what you are supposed to and failing miserably makes you
want to give up trying. As the commercial says, you may need
medication to help make it happen. But the whole diabetes thing
still makes you mad.

Most of us know when we are getting angry, at least in ret-
rospect. What usually happens is that we feel stress and tension begin to build in our body. If we miss this cue, maybe we
can realize that our breathing and heart rate and blood pressure
are increased (high blood pressure may cause a headache or your
face to flush). It is probably not a pretty sight and may even scare
our children and others we love. Looking in the mirror may help
us to calm down. I did not want anyone to remember me looking
like that. As weird as this may sound, anger can also drop your
blood sugar. Now that really takes the wind out of your sails and
stops you in mid-tirade as you run for the OJ!

The following are some more productive ways of dealing with
negative events in your life.

- Try to look back over the day and write things down that
  made you angry and/or frustrated. What time of day was
  it? How did you respond? Was your response productive?
  Did it solve the problem? If you can do this over a couple
  of weeks, you may begin to see a pattern. Does this always

seem to happen before lunch? Maybe it is a low blood sugar that made you respond that way. If you do have an episode of anger or frustration after lunch, maybe the cause is a high blood sugar. If you have a glucose meter, you can check it out at your next incident. Maybe your anger has nothing to do with blood sugar but more to do with the setting or the other people who set you off. If you can identify the situations and the people who make you angry you can plan better strategies ahead of time. Like everything else, you may have to experiment to see what works best for you. If you think you don't have time to do this, then continue experiencing your anger and frustration and see how unproductive it is. Some of this anger may come from your denial of your diabetes, feeling that you are weak and a failure because you have diabetes, or some other thing about yourself. Only if you analyze what is happening can you figure out what makes you mad and why.

- Think about how to calm yourself when you feel anger coming on. If your breathing is fast, work on slowing it down. Inhale deeply through your nose and exhale through pursed lips like you are blowing on a spoonful of soup. If you are sitting, go get a drink of water. If you are standing, sit down and lean back. If you are talking fast, slow down your speech by breathing in between each word. If your audience is looking at you like you have lost your mind, start laughing. It probably is very funny. I learned to focus on my boss's ears, which wiggled when she was reprimanding me for something. I tried not to smile, but this was harder than stopping my usual angry retort. I like using humor to defuse my anger, so that is often where I go. I collect books of jokes, books with funny titles or comical pictures, and I use visualization of the people who make me angry in ways that bring a smile to my face. Enough said. You get the picture.

- Find a way to take charge of your anger and make it productive, especially if it is your diabetes that is frustrating you and making you angry. Take one aspect of your diabetes care and work on it. The next time you are angry, go for a walk. You might find yourself walking faster and more energetically than you have ever done before. It will at least change the scene. Learn to be more assertive with people who try to tell you what to do about your diabetes. Prepare your speech ahead of time and practice delivering it out loud in front of a mirror so you will be prepared for the next encounter.

- Don't let a good "mad" go to waste. Use it as fuel. I started writing several books during angry fits. Some people draw or sketch, start dancing, sing as loud as they can in their car with the windows closed, or do something else creative that takes their mind off whatever made them angry. Change the target of your anger and express yourself without hurting anyone. When my boyfriend was in Vietnam, I realized I could not get mad at him in a letter. When I was angry with him, I taped his picture on the wall and threw a ball of Play-Doh at it. It really made me feel better.

Remember that anger can be an outward sign of depression, as it was with me, and you may need to see a therapist to help you unravel what is happening in your life and plan better strategies. Needing help and getting it is a sign of strength, not weakness. It affirms who you are and places you in control. When you seek help you are saying to yourself that you deserve to be helped and that you are worth helping.

STRESS

Having diabetes is certainly stressful. Sources of stress can also come from other physical illnesses and injuries. The mental challenges of depression, anger, and frustration discussed thus far definitely produce stress. Stress hormones are released in response to either physical or mental difficulties.

Stress moves your focus away from taking care of your health and diabetes. Long-term stress can also damage your cardiovascular system and cause stomach ulcers. This is true whether or not you have diabetes.

What Nurses Know...

Stress hormones, such as cortisol and adrenaline, cause an increase in blood pressure, pulse, and breathing rate as well as an increase in the release of stored glucose by the liver. This is very important in the fight-or-flight response but not useful when you really do not need to fight or run away.

All stress is not bad; whether it is good or bad depends on the level of stress we are experiencing. Mild stress levels are needed motivators of behavior. If we were not hungry, we might not get out of bed in the morning. Moderate concern over health issues may cause us to make or keep an appointment with our medical provider, work on a healthier diet, increase our exercise level, or monitor our blood sugar and blood pressure. However, high anxiety levels can be incapacitating. We have difficulty seeing the big picture because the stressor is so overwhelming. It makes conscious, logical thought very difficult and figuring out what to do about a situation next to impossible. Stress is also produced by happy events, as anyone getting married, having a baby, changing jobs, or making any other positively anticipated change in one's life can attest.

Everyone, regardless of whether they have diabetes, needs to learn how to manage situations before they become overwhelming. The following are some suggestions for coping with the stress in your life.

1. Indentify the stressor(s), such as rush hour traffic or a difficult coworker or boss.
2. Think about ways to avoid or minimize the occurrence(s). You might choose to leave home or work earlier or later, find

another route to or from work, apply for a transfer to a different department, or have a talk with your coworker or boss.

3. Change how you deal with stress, your coping style.
   - Ask yourself how else you can deal with the problem.
   - Talk yourself into accepting this problem as OK and maybe even beneficial.

4. Increase your physical activity. You may have to force yourself at first, but you may even look forward to it after awhile. If you don't use the energy produced by stress and anxiety, it will feed on itself and mushroom into something much bigger than it started out to be. So clean the bathroom or scrub the floor if you don't want to go for a walk, shoot hoops, or hit tennis balls against a backboard.

5. Develop creative outlets, such as those suggested in the "Anger and Frustration" section.

6. Decide to volunteer somewhere to help others and take the focus off of you and your problems. It does make you feel better.

7. Learn how to relax.

None of the following suggestions may come easily to you, but pick one and work at it until it becomes second nature:

- Breathing exercises: Sit in a comfortable chair or lie in bed and uncross your arms and legs. Breath in and out using your

What Nurses Know . . .

Stress blocks the release of insulin in type 2 diabetes, and some people may also be more sensitive to some of the stress hormones.

abdominal muscles and consciously relax your muscles every time you exhale. Do this for five to ten minutes or longer at least once a day.

- Progressive relaxation techniques: While continuing your slow breathing, contract and relax each group of muscles from your head to toes, or in the reverse order, until all of your muscles are relaxed. I described this technique more completely in Chapter 3. It is a great way to get yourself ready to sleep. You can also follow along with a CD on relaxation, but not while you are driving.
- Relaxation exercises: Take each joint and slowly move it through its full range of motion. Stretch each muscle individually as far as it will go. Follow a videotape or DVD to see how this is done, or see Chapter 3.
- Replace negative thoughts with positive ones. You need silence to do this. The younger you are, the more difficult this may seem for you. Most people today are bombarded with noise from the radio, iPod, cell phone, computer, and so on. *Turn them all off!* Close your door. Again, this may be uncomfortable, but after awhile you will get used to it and may even look forward to this period of silence in your busy life. Enjoy the silence while you breathe deeply and relax. When uncomfortable or negative thoughts invade this private moment, think of other, more positive ways to describe these thoughts or feelings or better responses to them. Think of something that makes you feel proud or happy, that makes you smile or laugh out loud.

If you want to get rid of stressful feelings you will have to work at any of the these techniques, because they probably represent something different than what you are doing now. Believe me, it is worth the effort. You will be developing strategies that you will use over and over again to get the upper hand on your multi-stress environment.

I talk about diabetes support groups in the next chapter, but let me recommend them here are well. In these groups, members tell their stories and respond to yours in positive ways. You can learn coping strategies from them and share some of your own. Unlike family and friends, they understand what you are dealing with and never tire of hearing what you have to say.

Positive Emotions

I have talked about replacing negative emotions with more uplifting and positive ones, so let me just describe some of these positive emotions and how they affect diabetes in general and blood glucose levels in particular.

Studies have shown that people with serious illnesses like diabetes who have a positive outlook on life live longer, perhaps because they have a healthier immune system. Researchers at the University of California at Irvine found that these positive people have lower levels of stress hormones and increased levels of growth hormones and beta-endorphins that reduce the effects of stress and strengthen the immune system. That doesn't mean that optimists have any less stress, anger, or frustration in their lives, or that they were born into wonderful, supportive, and loving families and were raised by very positive and nurturing parents. They were not necessarily *lucky*. Instead, most learned how to think differently about negative events in their lives and how to learn from these occurrences. They learned to be their own best friends by looking for and valuing their own attributes. They realized that positive emotions, such as love, joy, happiness, hope, gratitude, and so on, help them to thrive and grow as a person, and they valued that. They learned that how they talked to themselves could be damaging to their ability to cope or be uplifting and could enhance their quality of life, and they consciously chose the latter. Some may have been blessed with a sunny outlook, but most worked at changing, associating with positive people, and learning not to take themselves too seriously. What are the alternatives? I don't know about you, but feeling sorry for myself or bad-mouthing myself has never made me happy or inspired me to work on changing the mess I have occasionally found myself in.

What does being more optimistic and positive do to blood sugars? If you are having difficulties with high blood glucose levels even two or three hours after a meal, maybe the problem isn't what you ate but how much you found to laugh about. A study in Japan with people who had type 2 diabetes and were not on insulin showed that when these people watched a comedy show after a meal they had lower two-hour postprandial glucose levels than those same people who ate a similar meal but then attended a lecture without anything to laugh about. The researchers explained that laughter may have accelerated glucose use by increasing the muscular activity used in laughing, or that the positive emotions acted against the hormones that help to increase blood sugars after a meal. Wow! Now all we need to do is find something to keep us laughing.

As I watched my own children growing up, and now watch my three-year-old grandsons playing, it has occurred to me how joyous and gleeful they are and how much they love life. (Unless, of course they are hungry, tired, or have realized what buttons they can push to get a rise out of us. Yes, my children and grandchildren are normal.) Having children around should make us smile and even laugh out loud when we hear the giggling, even if we don't know what they are laughing about. In fact, if you knew, you may not find it funny. If you don't have your own children or grandchildren to teach you how to laugh, go to a park, or volunteer for the church nursery.

There are professionals such as humor therapists whose job it is to help people learn to laugh and take themselves less seriously. Some suggestions they have include scheduling funny things in your life, such as a movie, TV show, or a funny radio program like *A Prairie Home Companion* with Garrison Keillor or *Car Talk* with the Tappet Brothers. Listening to a funny book on a CD on your way to work or when coming home, or both, will at least put a smile on your face and set you up for a more positive outlook on your day. Read the comics in the newspaper or online and cut out strips that you identify with. Post them on your refrigerator, bulletin board, office door, or computer. Learn to laugh at yourself when you pull an "oops," and everyone will think you did it on purpose. If you don't have a joke book, get one. If you have one, when was the last time you read it? This is serious healthful business! It is called *chuckle therapy* by those whose job it is to know. So go have a belly laugh and call it exercise. Your clothes might fit better in the morning.

Find positive, optimistic people to be around, and learn to become one for them. When I am saying something negative my daughter will remind me not to be a "Debbie Downer." That is our signal to each other to lighten up. We cannot be upbeat all the time! If the people in your life are more negative than positive, limit your exposure to them, read about support groups in Chapter 9, or have those people read Chapter 10.

Dealing with depression; anger; frustration; and situations that make you want to cry, smash things, or run and hide, added to living with diabetes, can be difficult. Most of us need help, and sometimes medication. Doing nothing should not be an option. Stress can be debilitating and raise blood sugar, but it does not have to. Attitude is everything, so if you need a push in the right direction, consider this chapter as my boot in the pants. Get going. You can be successful at changing your circumstance like anyone else... if *you* choose to.

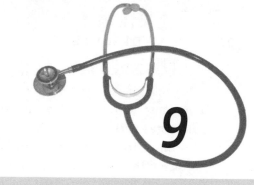

9

How Can I Get the Help I Need?

I've had type 1 diabetes since I was two years old. My mother did a good job helping me control blood sugars while I was growing up, but when I got my first job after high school and had to use a doctor approved by the group insurance, I got into trouble. She didn't seem to understand about type 1 diabetes and told me that I could get off insulin if I just ate right and exercised. She was blaming me for my poor control! She gave me no information so I could eat better, and she did not do any lab work the whole two years I went to her. I didn't even see her on every visit, but the other doctors there were no better. I stopped seeing anyone for my diabetes until I came here. This was the first time I had an A1c done, and it was 15%!   HENRY

Some of you with type 1 or type 2 diabetes can relate to Henry in that your healthcare practitioner blamed you for your uncontrolled blood sugars even if you were doing everything you knew to do. You may have even been called a *noncompliant patient* because of your high glucose levels. You received no or minimal instructions on diet and exercise, and your precious fifteen minutes with your healthcare practitioner was spent doing an exam, writing out a prescription, ordering tests, and ushering you out the door so the next patient could come in. You never got to ask questions or, if you did, you got some vague answer that didn't really help. You never got to tell your story. Someone else took your history, or you filled out a history form and the person treating your diabetes never seemed to know what was in it. How is that going to help you as an individual try to control this all-encompassing disease? Your frustration is justified, and in this chapter I list the criteria of a healthcare professional that you should hire as your medical provider and how to find one that works for you. Yes, I said *hire*, because that is exactly what you are doing. You (or your insurance plus your copay) pays his or her salary, so you ought to get your money's worth! In this book I use the word *client* instead of *patient* to talk about a person with diabetes, because the former indicates that you have the power to hire and fire your healthcare provider. It makes you part of the team working to improve and maintain diabetes control. As a *client* you should feel not only empowered but also responsible for your own actions concerning blood glucose control and diabetes *self*-management. You must learn all you can about diabetes and the effects of food, exercise, and medication on blood sugar control with the help and guidance of a healthcare practitioner who includes you in the decision-making process. The best laid plans are useless if they don't take into account your situation and your needs. Therefore, you must be part of the healthcare team no matter how scary that may seem to you.

We know our bodies best, and we need to learn how to take care of ourselves with lots of help from others. Lorig and Halsted listed six self-management skills we need to learn how to do:

1. *Problem-solving skills* start with identifying the problems we face. Maybe they are financial or psychological or physical.

With help, we can make a list of possible solutions, such as how to pay for the medications listed in Chapter 4, seeing a counselor or therapist for the emotional or family issues discussed in Chapters 8 and 10, or getting a referral to a medical provider who can assist with physical limitations or the beginning symptoms of a complication. We then must act on these suggestions and evaluate the results. Did the suggestions work?

2. *Decision making* is the next skill to learn. We must have enough information to decide what to eat and when to eat, whether to exercise or not based on our blood sugars, and to understand our medication so we can evaluate whether it is working the way it should to control glucose levels. Many of us make countless decisions about our diabetes each and every day, and we must be trained to do so effectively.

3. *Finding and using available resources* is the next skill needed for diabetes self-management. This chapter lists some resources you may need. There is also a long list of resources in the back of this book. You must have the courage and fortitude to do the research and make the call.

4. *Forming a partnership with your healthcare provider or diabetes educator* is an essential skill. You need to trust this person enough to share with him or her what is really happening in your life. You have to be honest and give specifics of how diabetes affects you, what is working and what is not working, or what needs to change. How else can he or she give you the specific information and help you need? Keep looking until you find the right person for you.

5. *Taking aim at diabetes control and taking action* will help you overcome the difficulties you encounter, no mater how big or small. You may never have thought of yourself as a person who can stand up and be counted, who can step up to the plate and hit the ball, but your quality of life, and even your life itself, may depend on it.

6. The last skill you must learn in this diabetes self-management educational process is how to *self-tailor what you learn to how*

you and your body react to anything that you try. Only you can make the critical decisions as to what you do with the information you are getting. For some people this may be frightening. It was for me in the beginning, but after awhile it made sense. It then became very empowering.

So who are the people with whom you can partner to learn what you need to know to deal with this disease? Start with a diabetes educator.

Diabetes Educators

Because diabetes is such a complex disease, it takes a team of diabetes educators and other professionals to really provide the care you need even if you "only" have type 2 diabetes. These dedicated healthcare professionals can come from a number of disciplines. Throughout this book I have referred to *healthcare providers* and *healthcare practitioners* instead of *doctors* because these individuals may not be MDs. The American Diabetes Association (ADA), in its 2010 *Standards of Medical Care in Diabetes,* stated that "Diabetes self-management education (DSME) is an on-going process of facilitating the knowledge, skill, and ability necessary for diabetes self-care....The overall objectives of DSME are to support informed decision-making, self-care behaviors, problem-solving, and active collaboration with the health care team and to improve clinical outcomes, health status, and quality of life in a cost-effective manner." Most states have laws that require insurance companies to pay for diabetes education, but you need to know how to find a diabetes educator who can provide this vital information. Go to the American Association of Diabetes Educators' Web site, www.aadenet.org, click on "Find a Diabetes Educator," and put in your zip code or click on your state. You will get a list of certified diabetes educators (CDEs) in your area. They are mainly nurses (RNs), nurse practitioners (NPs) or advanced practice nurses (APRNs), registered dieticians (RDs), and pharmacists (RPhs or PharmDs). Many of the RNs, NPs, and APRNs work with internists and endocrinologists. They see clients in their offices, hospitals, managed care organizations, home healthcare, clinics, and other settings. RDs and pharmacists see clients were they work. Most diabetes educators have master's degrees or higher in their discipline and have passed a difficult certification exam that they must retake every five years, or participate in relevant continuing education activities. This keeps them up to date on all current information, medication, and components of teaching diabetes self-management. Diabetes educators give people with diabetes the knowledge, skills, and tools they need to successfully manage their diabetes and avoid many of the complications associated with the disease.

This sounds like a comprehensive approach to helping you learn about how to manage your diabetes. If you agree, find a diabetes educator and make an appointment.

You may already be seeing an internist or an endocrinologist for your three- to six-month checkups, or you may be followed by a nurse diabetes educator and see a doctor only when things

What Nurses Know ...

Diabetes educators teach and monitor the seven self-care behaviors that help you improve your health status and quality of life. These behaviors include:

- Eating a healthy diet
- Being more active
- Monitoring blood sugar levels
- Taking medication appropriately
- Problem solving when blood glucose is too high or too low
- Coping with life's challenges in a healthy way
- Reducing the risks for hyper- and hypoglycemia and long-term complications

What Nurses Know...

Telling your story might be the best thing that ever happened to you. The result is that you will get a very individualized plan of care tailored to your needs, both financial and emotional, and your fears about medication, exercise, food preferences, and needed lifestyle changes.

are not going well. I can assure you that a diabetes educator can and will spend the time it takes to help you get a handle on your situation.

An NP can prescribe medications in most states, so discuss your medications with her or him. He or she may adjust the dose, change the medication, or suggest other ways that you can use these medications to help control your blood glucose levels.

At the beginning of this book I talk about writing down your questions on an ongoing basis. Keep a magnetic pad on the front of your refrigerator or computer with a pencil or pen attached, and write questions down when something occurs to you. Take this list to your next appointment with the diabetes educator. If you need a lot of time for discussion, schedule a longer appointment so you will not feel rushed. Prioritize your questions so if there is not enough time you will get your most important questions answered. Then be prepared to do your homework and follow through with what you and your diabetes educator decide.

Two other practitioners who are also diabetes educators are RDs and pharmacists. They also want and need to have client contact to keep their certification credentials. Find each in your area and make an appointment. An RD can be invaluable in helping you make a meal plan that takes into consideration your likes and dislikes, within reason. If you don't do the grocery shopping or the cooking, take along to the appointment the person in your house who does. Besides, two heads are always better than one. You can learn more at www.mydiabetespartner.org. If you are confused about your medication, or about drug and food interactions, make an appointment with your pharmacist or find one who is also a diabetes educator. Again take your questions and the list of all of your medications, supplements, and over-the-counter drugs for any and all sporadic occurrences so he or she can evaluate your situation and make recommendations that work for you. If you are having difficulty paying for your meds, the pharmacist can direct you to services that can help or see if a cheaper generic drug can be substituted. You are not alone. There are many health-care practitioners who have the training, the ability, and the desire to help you learn this diabetes self-management stuff. If you are turned off by anyone, look for another diabetes educator who is more to your liking.

Support Groups

Another big help for me was my support group. Contact the ADA chapter in your area to locate one or to attend meetings and workshops that might put you in contact with others who are working at diabetes control like you. I went to everything I could find about diabetes in the early years and started a support group at the end of one of these workshops. Start by joining the ADA chapter near you and go to meetings. For $28 a year (2010 rate) you get *Diabetes Forecast*, the best journal for people with diabetes and their family I have ever read. Look at previews of the current issue at www.forecast.diabetes.org and see for yourself. Sign up to get on the list of people to be contacted when something related to diabetes education is planned. You can also sign up to receive e-mails from the ADA chapter at your home or work computer. Let your family and friends know you want to join. This membership could be the best Christmas or birthday gift they have ever given you.

Speaking of family and friends, their support can be vital to your successful control of blood glucose levels. Such support is a great help to anyone with a chronic illness, and those of us with diabetes are no exception. I knew a man who had type 1 diabetes and had just returned from an African safari. I was impressed that he would do something so adventurous while carrying insulin, syringes, his meter and test strips, and all of the rest of the diabetes paraphernalia, so he showed me the miniature case that he put it all in. I then asked if his companions on the trip knew how to help him if he got in trouble and he said that no one on this trip knew he had diabetes. The only person he had ever confided in was his wife and she did not accompany him. In fact, none of his coworkers or tennis or golf partners knew he had diabetes, and he was proud of that fact. He was either very brave or very stupid, and I wished him luck, because he was going to need it. Protecting your privacy and your health may be mutually exclusive. Most of your family and friends have your best interest at heart but may not know what they can do to help. You may need to make suggestions, especially if someone becomes the "food police" and tries to tell you what you can and cannot eat due to their excessive but uninformed concern about your health, or you encounter a "dessert pusher" who feels sorry for you and suggests that you can have a little piece since they made a treat just for you. If these people are important to you, don't avoid them. Teach them what they need to know about your diabetes, the healthy diet you are trying to follow, and what else you are doing to help normalize your blood sugars. Tell them what they can say or do that will help you to follow the program you and your diabetes educator have formulated. Ask them to read Chapter 10 of this book. It was written for them. You may even want to invite them to come with you to your next healthcare appointment and encourage them to bring their own list of questions. The next time you are with them, take control of the situation by choosing the restaurant (after going online to preselect an appropriate entree or two) or bring a low-calorie, low-carb dessert to share at the next office party or family gathering. There are many options in cookbooks and on the Web. When I bring a treat to a social or work get-together there is usually nothing left to take home. It seems everyone is trying to lose weight, and my friends and coworkers know that what I bring will taste good and help them to do that. Now I take copies of the recipe for those who ask.

You need to trust some people with the information about your diabetes and teach them what they need to know that might save your life. As you work at controlling your blood sugar, blood pressure, and cholesterol with diet, exercise, and maybe medication, you can at least gain their admiration and might even teach *them* how to live a healthier lifestyle. After all, the controls I have discussed so far are not just for those of us with diabetes.

Other Healthcare Practitioners

There are several other healthcare professionals you should see at least on a yearly basis.

A periodontist, or a really good dentist knowledgeable about diabetes and gum disease, is a must, because checking for gum disease is an ongoing process and must be done at least yearly, if not every six months. A thorough removal of plaque deposits around the teeth and gums is a necessary measure to prevent gingivitis and periodontitis. Some of us are more prone to these

What Nurses Know . . .

The periodontist will need a list of your medications, both prescription and over the counter; as well as supplements; herbal remedies; and any meds you may take for occasional pain, gas, nausea, constipation, or diarrhea. Also provide a history of allergies.

problems than others based on family history and control of blood glucose levels. If problems develop, your dentist may want to see you every three or four months.

If teeth grinding is a problem, you may need a mouth guard to wear at night to protect your teeth from excessive wear and chipping. If financial concerns are a problem, see if there is a medical center near where you live that offers free exams and treatment at their dental school. There are also clinics staffed by volunteer dentists and dental hygienists who offer dental care for free or on a sliding fee basis if you meet the criteria. You also can check the Health Resources and Services Administration's Web site, www.hrsa.gov, for a list of affordable healthcare centers.

Seeing an ophthalmologist who is a retinal specialist is a must every year to check on the health of your retinas. If you are developing retinopathy, dilated pupillary exams may be needed every three to four months, and laser treatments of fragile blood vessels to prevent bleeding into the back of the eye may be needed. This care may also be found at a local medical center.

Podiatrists are doctors of podiatric medicine (DPMs) and also are known as *podiatric physicians* or *podiatric surgeons.* They are qualified by their education and training to diagnose and treat conditions affecting the foot, ankle, and related

What Nurses Know...

Treating corns, calluses, ingrown toenails, or other foot ailments should never be done by you with over-the-counter preparations that could cause skin trauma and difficulty healing, even if you do not have peripheral artery disease. Consult your healthcare professional to determine the best treatment options.

structures of the leg. You may need to see a podiatrist if you have any problems with your feet even if the issues are not related to diabetes.

If you have any problem seeing well enough to cut your toenails safely, a podiatrist should do this every two to three months or as needed to prevent inadvertent cutting of the skin or causing an ingrown toenail that could possibly lead to infection. The nearest medical center can direct you to a clinic or office that takes reduced or no fees, or check the American Podiatric Medical Association's home page at www.apma.org and click on "Find a Podiatrist."

You may need to see a psychologist if and when you have emotional issues that are complicating your diabetes control. If you need medication for depression or other emotional problems, a psychologist can call your healthcare provider to get one, because psychologists in most states do not have prescriptive authority. Ask your diabetes educator for a referral, or go to the psychologist locator run by the American Psychological Association Practice Organization at http://locator.apa.org to find one in your area.

If you have started to develop complications you may need to see the following medical care providers:

- A *cardiologist* should at least be consulted if you have evidence of plaque buildup in coronary arteries or any symptoms of angina.
- A *vascular surgeon* would follow any cholesterol plaque buildup in carotid arteries and peripheral artery disease to assess when an intervention may be necessary.
- A *nephrologist* should care for any kidney-related problems.
- A *neurologist* may be needed to follow any development of nerve damage anywhere in the body.
- Seeing a *urologist* or an *obstetrician/gynecologist* for sexual dysfunction problems may become necessary.
- *Physical and occupational therapists* are indispensable for any problems related to a stroke or painful joints. They can teach you exercises to increase range of motion and make it

easier to do some activities of daily living, such as using utensils and buttoning clothing.

What I wanted most as a newly diagnosed diabetic was a set of rules to help me live with this chronic illness. As I left the doctor's office that day of my diagnosis, I wondered what in the world I could fix for dinner that evening. Because I was never an inpatient, I did not have the luxury of having a consultation with a registered dietitian, so I bought a diabetic cookbook. By dinnertime I had decided that what we usually ate was going to have to do. At my next office visit, I asked to see a dietitian and was told my insurance would not cover this as an outpatient. I told my doctor that he had two choices: He could teach me what I needed to know about my diet, or he could request a dietary consult. So for the grand total of $16 an hour I sat with first one, then a second registered dietitian, learned the standard instruction, and then picked their brains for rationale and "what ifs" and got my questions answered. It occurred to me then that if I had not insisted on getting someone to teach me what I needed to know, I might still be floundering and overwhelmed. The second thing that occurred to me after this experience was that the rest of my education was up to me. What a scary thought, but at least I had a head start.

After about a year and a half into my career as a diabetic, a wonderful thing happened. I was asked, along with many others with type 1 and type 2 diabetes, to participate in a research project to see if diabetics could be trained to be better guessers of blood sugars, both high and low. At that point glucose monitors were just becoming popular and affordable (but not small and not covered by insurance yet). I jumped at the opportunity. Toward the end of the 6 weeks, the participants and I were communicating with each other more than the researchers were. I asked if the other participants wanted to continue to meet as a support group. The response was overwhelming. Because I needed a support group and there was none in my area, I started one. I led this group for 7 years, well after it had met my personal needs. I learned how desperate people and their families were for any advice, education, and opportunities to share their stories. This all came about by dumb luck, but if it weren't for dumb luck, some of us would have no luck at all. And some of us may need to make our own luck by contacting the right healthcare practitioners that we need at the time.

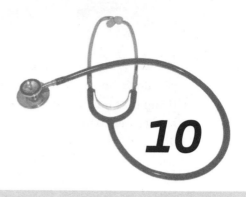

10

How Can Family and Friends Help?

My son is very overweight and falls asleep after dinner. I worry that he has diabetes but he won't see a doctor. What can I do to help? IVAN

My friend has type 1 diabetes, and I have tried to tell her what my Internet sources say about how she can get off insulin, but she won't listen. What else can I say to her? JACKIE

When I told my brother I had diabetes, he sarcastically thanked me for adding yet another hereditary disease to our family medical history. That reaction was worse than my diagnosis. It added guilt to everything else I was feeling. SUE

If you recognize yourself in any of the above vignettes, this chapter was written for you. You have a loved one, friend, or coworker who has diabetes and you want to be helpful but you don't know what to say or do. Maybe you have said something that has made the person with diabetes angry or caused him or her to avoid you. If you want to demonstrate your support for this person, there are several things you can do and some that you should not do or say. First of all, diabetes is a complex disease and difficult to control. People with diabetes want and need your support. If you have read the beginning of this book, you know that I have type 1 diabetes and am a diabetes educator. Even though my friends, coworkers, and family members know this, I still get unsolicited advice and inappropriate dietary suggestions. If this happens to me, then it must happen to others with diabetes. To family, friends, and coworkers: We all know that you love us, worry about us, and want only the best for us. However, this is what we want you to realize:

- We are all different, and the way we experience diabetes and treat it is different.
- We are not perfect, and even though we do a good job of handling our symptoms and controlling blood sugars, unexpected things happen.
- Low blood sugar or high blood sugar can make us grouchy and difficult to live with.
- We are not *diabetics* unless we choose to call ourselves that. We are people first who happen to have diabetes.
- We are the same people we were before being diagnosed with diabetes, so don't treat us differently than you did before. If we have changed at all, maybe we are a little smarter since we have learned so much because of the diagnosis.
- Try to put yourself in our position and think about what you might want us to say or do that would be helpful to you.
- We don't want your pity. We want and need your *support*. Ask us about diabetes or how we are doing. It might surprise you that we are trying to live a healthy lifestyle, the same lifestyle that you are, or should be, living.

There is a difference between type 1 and type 2 diabetes, and age does not define what type you have. I was almost 40 when I developed type 1. This usually happens in childhood, but obviously not always, and there are children and teenagers who are diagnosed with type 2 diabetes, which is no longer reserved for adults. Type 1 diabetes is always treated with insulin for life, and some people with type 2 also need insulin to control blood sugars. This is something Jackie in the second vignette at the beginning of this chapter needs to learn. Needing insulin does not mean diabetes is getting worse. Type 1 isn't the "bad" kind, and type 2 is much more than a "touch of sugar." Both can lead to complications, but that is by no means a forgone conclusion. Reading Chapter 1 of this book may help you to understand the differences between type 1 and type 2 diabetes and how they are treated.

Food issues are typically of concern to family and friends as well as those of us with diabetes. Get a diabetes cookbook, or find recipes online at www.dlife.com, www.diabetes.org, or just search for diabetes and recipes. Do not be surprised if a person with diabetes asks you about the ingredients in your food so he or she can decide how much to eat or how much insulin he or she needs to give. People with diabetes *can* eat sugar. It is a carb just

What Nurses Know...

The more you know about diabetes, symptoms of low and high blood sugars and how to treat them, the carbohydrate values of various foods, and how exercise affects blood sugar, the better you can support your friend or family member who has diabetes. Read the earlier chapters in this book, or go online to get more information.

like fruit, milk, bread, starchy vegetables, and flour. All of these contribute to raising blood sugar; however, they are all part of a healthy diet and should be eaten in moderation. If you use a cookbook that has nutritional values per serving size, the number of carbohydrates and how many servings are in the recipe are important pieces of information for people who are counting carbs.

Some people who don't have diabetes become the "diabetes police" and say things like "You can't eat that. It has sugar in it." or "What is your blood sugar? Isn't that too high?" These comments are viewed as attempts to take control from the only person who should have control: the person who has diabetes. Saying things like this indicates that you do not trust that he or she can or will make good judgments about how to control blood sugars. If you serve healthy foods, let the person choose what and how much to eat, like anyone else. If you don't serve healthy foods, don't be surprised if your friend or relative brings some to share. Some people also become "dessert pushers" and say things like "Just have a little piece. I made it just for you." This comes across as feeling sorry for the person with diabetes, who can't eat the *good* stuff anymore, poor thing.

Your loved ones may have fluctuations in blood sugars through no fault of their own. There are so many issues that affect glucose levels, such as emotions, other medications, infections, and other medical conditions that are common to people without diabetes as well, so it is hard to always be in control. If this person acts differently toward you or seems angry or listless and confused, it may be related to that person's blood sugar. Ask what you can do to help, from getting some orange juice, encouraging him or her to test blood sugar, or simply doing nothing. If the person with diabetes is not forthcoming with information and you are truly worried, feel his or her skin. Low blood sugar will produce cool and clammy skin, whereas with high blood sugar the skin will be warm and dry. After the episode, ask about what he or she would like you to do in the future so you can be prepared.

What Nurses Know...

The following are tips for helping a person with diabetes management.

1. *Learn about diabetes. Read the first five chapters of this book, go to the American Diabetes Association's Web site (www.diabetes.org), or search online for information. Always put the current year after the search term (e.g., diabetes 2010) so the up-to-date information will be listed first.*

2. *Ask the person with diabetes about how he or she experiences diabetes.*

3. *Ask how you can help. Ask the person to tell you anything you do or say that makes life with diabetes more difficult for him or her. If this person does not give specifics, at least you have indicated your interest in knowing.*

4. *If what you are doing or saying seems to irritate or make maters worse, try something new. More of the same is not going to work any better.*

5. *Get help for both of you. Find a support group and go with or without the person who has diabetes. Look for a local chapter of the American Diabetes Association in the phone book and call.*

If you are like Ivan in the first vignette at the beginning of this chapter and are concerned that your loved one is not taking care of himself, all you can do is tell him of your concern and demonstrate your love for him by saying that you want to be supportive if and when he needs you to be. It is very hard for a parent or sibling to see an adult family member not take care of himself, but there is nothing more you can do until that person is ready.

Nagging will only make him resentful and want to avoid you. Leading by example might help. You can live a healthy lifestyle; serve or choose appropriate foods at home or at a restaurant; and walk more, inviting this person to join you. You can also ask, in a nonthreatening way, why he or she is not seeing a healthcare provider or following the regimen prescribed. The reason may be something you can help with, from finding a low- or no-cost means of covering medical care and medication to listening to his fear that a hereditary medical condition might be diagnosed. Again, offering your support and encouragement is important. Going with your loved one to see the healthcare provider may also be helpful. As hard as this may be to realize, it may take a trip to the emergency room to be a wake-up call for him or her. You can't make that person take personal care and responsibility for his actions until he or she is ready.

As Sue found out in the third vignette, there is a lot of guilt involved with the diagnosis of diabetes. Because diabetes is usually a hereditary illness, relatives want to know where it came from. Since there was no one in my family with diabetes, which is often the case with type 1 diabetes, my own mother blamed it on my deceased father's side. What does it really matter and how is this helpful? People diagnosed with diabetes often blame themselves for this disease. Eating too much sugar did not cause diabetes. There is no shame in being diagnosed with diabetes so there should be no guilt. It was the luck of the draw and now we must all learn to deal with it in the best way possible.

Accentuate the positive. When I was freaking out about my diagnosis and what it might mean for me and my family's future, my husband hugged me and reassured me that we would tackle this together. He had faith in me and my ability to learn what I needed to know and do what I needed to so I could control this disease. He reminded me of my successes in the past and that this was but another challenge that I would overcome. There was no pity in his eyes or look of fear as to how it would impact him. He even went with me to several workshops offered by the

American Diabetes Association so he could learn all he could and make good on his promise to work with me. I recently asked my now grown children if they worried about getting diabetes. Both reassured me that they felt if it happened, they could deal with it as I had. Even after 25 years, I still need all the pats on the back I can get.

Here are 10 examples of *Diabetes Etiquette* devised by William Polonski of the Behavioral Diabetes Institute. You can find a printable list at http://behavioraldiabetesinstitute.org/downloads/Etiquette-Card.pdf and more information at http://behavioraldiabetesinstitute.org. My copy is posted on my refrigerator.

DO'S AND DON'TS OF DIABETES ETIQETTE

DON'T offer unsolicited advice about my eating or other aspects of diabetes. You may mean well, but giving advice about someone's personal habits, especially when it is not requested, isn't very nice. Besides, many of the popularly held beliefs about diabetes ("you should just stop eating sugar") are out of date or just plain wrong.

DO realize and appreciate that diabetes is hard work. Diabetes management is a full-time job that I didn't apply for, didn't want, and can't quit. It involves thinking about what, when, and how much I eat, while also factoring in exercise, medication, stress, blood sugar monitoring, and so much more – each and every day.

DON'T tell me horror stories about your grandmother or other people with diabetes you have heard about. Diabetes is scary enough, and stories like these are not reassuring! Besides, we now know that with good management, odds are good you can live a long, healthy, and happy life with diabetes.

DO offer to join me in making healthy lifestyle changes. Not having to be alone with efforts to change, like starting an exercise program, is one of the most powerful ways that you can be helpful. After all, healthy lifestyle changes can benefit everyone!

DON'T look so horrified when I check my blood sugars or give myself an injection. It is not a lot of fun for me either. Checking blood sugars and taking medications are things I must do to manage diabetes well. If I have to hide while I do so, it makes it much harder for me.

(Continued)

DO ask how you might be helpful. If you want to be supportive, there may be lots of little things I would probably appreciate your help with. However, what I really need may be very different than what you think I need, so please ask first.

DON'T offer thoughtless reassurances. When you first learn about my diabetes, you may want to reassure me by saying things like, "Hey it could be worse; you could have cancer!" This won't make me feel better. And the implicit message seems to be that diabetes is no big deal. However, diabetes (like cancer) IS a big deal.

DO be supportive of my efforts for self-care. Help me set up an environment for success by supporting healthy food choices. Please honor my decision to decline a particular food, even when you really want me to try it. You are most helpful when you are not being a source of unnecessary temptation.

DON'T peek at or comment on my blood glucose numbers without asking me first. These numbers are private unless I choose to share them. It is normal to have numbers that are sometimes too low or too high. Your unsolicited comments about these numbers can add to the disappointment, frustration and anger I already feel.

DO offer your love and encouragement. As I work hard to manage diabetes successfully, sometimes just knowing that you care can be very helpful and motivating.

Reprinted from *Diabetes Etiquette*, a booklet written by William H. Polonsky and staff at the Behavioral Diabetes Institute with permission from William H. Polonsky.

Of course the reverse can also be a problem. Some people with diabetes are not very considerate of others who don't have it. If there is anything that your family member or friend does that makes you uncomfortable like making a big deal about injecting insulin in front of you or making rude comments about what you choose to serve for dinner, please speak up. We all should be considerate of each other. This disease also impacts those of you who love us. By sharing with each other our concerns openly and honestly, we can learn from each other and grow stronger together. By being patient with each other, we can deal with how this disease affects us all.

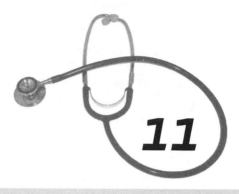

11

Staying Motivated

I sometimes get discouraged and want to give up. I lose weight and gain it back. My A1c is not coming down the way my doctor wants it to. How do I stay motivated to continue to do what I know I should? MARY

I knew a man who was recently diagnosed with type 2 diabetes and could not tolerate the medication that was prescribed, so he stopped taking it. He did what he thought he was supposed to do to control his blood glucose levels but was failing miserably. Like Mary, he wanted to give up. He had stopped monitoring his blood sugar because the numbers were too high and he did not want to see them. One day, his glucose was 205 mg/dl, and he was very discouraged. He feared he was going to be put on insulin, a common fear that many have because they dread injections. When I told him that if he ate a healthy diet (reinforced by a handout on carb counting, portion control, and nonfrying cooking methods) and lost ten to twenty pounds, he might not need any medication, he was energized and willing to try. He thought exercise was not a problem because he stocked shelves at a grocery store all night, but he was willing to get a pedometer to see exactly how much he did walk. And he was not only willing to test his blood sugars again but also willing to record them, along with what he ate, in a booklet I gave him. The plan we came up with had him losing five to ten pounds by his next visit and bringing in his booklet so we could talk about the blood sugar numbers and his food choices. He was given a prescription for a different medication until his blood glucose level came down. What motivated him was getting off medication and staying off insulin.

Getting motivated to make changes in your life is difficult for everyone. Anyone who has lost weight knows this regardless of whether diabetes is the reason. Making the commitment to do something different is the first step to achieving success. Finding the tools to begin the process is the second step. These tools may include researching a weight-loss program that you think might work for you; joining a gym or getting a personal trainer to help you with exercise; buying an exercise CD or weights for use at home; finding time in your overcrowded schedule to walk and keep track of food intake, either manually or on the computer; getting a glucose meter and buying strips even if you have to pay out-of-pocket for them; and finding the professional help you need to accomplish your goals (see Chapter 9 for relevant suggestions).

By reading this book, or at least parts of it, you have demonstrated that you are now ready for the third step: setting goals. Make a list of desired outcomes (goals), from weight loss to increasing physical activity to decreasing your A1c. Make these goals as specific as possible, or you will not get around to it; reasonable and realistic, or you will fail and get discouraged; and, most important, personal. These goals should not be what your health care practitioner has outlined (unless you agree with him or her). I specifically told my current healthcare team on my first visit that unless I brought it up, I did not want to be harassed with a discussion about losing weight. My stated goal was to normalize blood sugars without experiencing frequent lows. If in the process I lost weight and increased my exercise level, we would all celebrate. That was fifteen years ago. I would have found another medical practice if my informed wishes were not respected.

Your family or loved ones may have their own goals for you. Their goals may not be your goals, so you need to set them straight about what *you* want to accomplish. I am sure my husband hated getting up in the middle of the night to get me orange juice when I had my frequent hypoglycemic episodes, at times four or five nights per week. He never complained because he realized I was doing my best to normalize my blood glucose levels. However, I'm sure he loves my insulin pump as much as I do because I rarely wake him up anymore. If family or friends annoy you with this or that suggestion, talk to them about how unhelpful this is and explain how angry it makes you. Have a signal when they are crossing the line (like saying "Zip it," or indicating as much by putting your fingers across your lips or any other explained reaction to their perceived interference). There is a funny commercial in which a mother tries to stop the supermarket clerk from talking about the serving of vegetables in Chef Boyardee ravioli in front of her school-age child. You don't have to knock over a pyramid of cans (as the mom does in the commercial) to make your point. Just practice some of her facial expressions. You should realize that your family and friends are only human and usually only want the best for you. Their comments are motivated more by fear or a lack of understanding or denial that there is anything wrong with you than a malicious desire to undermine your goals. So, depending on why you think they are doing what they are doing, try to reassure or explain or, better yet, ask them to accompany you on your next visit to your health care practitioner. Another potential solution is to have them read Chapter 10, which was written for family and friends, so they can learn how to better express their concern or be more supportive. Be sure to highlight the part that pertains to them or the part that would be most helpful to you. Another resource is www.dlife.com, which contains more helpful suggestions. Sign up for their free newsletter on the right-hand side of their home page.

What Nurses Know...

Steps to get motivated include the following:

1. *Make a commitment to change by saying aloud or writing down your resolve to do whatever it takes to live a healthier lifestyle.*
2. *Find the resources you think you need to learn how to do this and to help you remain accountable. These tools will depend on the goal(s) you choose.*
3. *Make a written list of goals you wish to achieve. Prioritize them from most important (to you) to least. Make them*

   - *specific (how much weight loss, increase in activity, decrease in A1c, etc.);*
   - *reasonable, realistic, and achievable (one- to two-pound loss per week, a ten-minute increase in exercise per week, decrease your A1c by 0.5% or 0.25% by your next visit); and*
   - *personal (what matters most to you, from feeling better and using fewer sick days, to losing a clothing size, etc).*

4. *Find a role model to inspire you, from a celebrity to a family member or an acquaintance.*
5. *Set a start date and make it soon, like tomorrow or next Monday. Write it on the calendar with a big star or bold it—no excuses, ready or not.*

Attitude is Everything

If all you see in your future is doom and gloom because you have diabetes, then you will not work at controlling your blood sugars, losing weight, or becoming more active. You will not feel very good physically as your blood glucose levels go higher and higher. You'll get sick a lot more, because hyperglycemia depresses your immune system. Emotionally, you may feel defeated and get depressed about your circumstances. You'll define yourself as a diabetic (sickly) and play the "ain't it awful" game, first described by Eric Berne 40 years ago in *Games People Play.* People may seem sorry for you for awhile but will soon become weary of the drain you have on their emotions and will start to avoid you if they can. Do you really want that?

Another game that some people who are diagnosed with a chronic illness play is the "yes, but..." game. After reading or hearing advice on controlling diabetes, they might say out loud or internally something like "Yes, that sounds great, but it will never work because..." This is another form of "ain't it awful." It gives a person the excuse to avoid responsibility. In other words, it provides a reason not to change or work at controlling the disease process. People who do this think things like "If I'm going to get complications and die early anyway, why bother? What is the point? Yes, but..." If either of the preceding scenarios describes you, WAKE UP! You, and only you, can make a huge difference and change everything, but first you need an attitude adjustment.

Find a role model. There are plenty of celebrities, athletes, and important people to choose from who have either type 1 or type 2 diabetes. Again, dLife features some of these people regularly on its Web site. They are extraordinary in spite of their diabetes and sometimes because of their diabetes. One name that has been in the news lately is Bret Michaels, a recent Celebrity Apprentice winner, rock musician, singer, front man for the band Poison, and a type 1 diabetic since childhood. He never let his diabetes get in the way of what he wanted out of life, despite several medical emergencies while he participated in Celebrity Apprentice.

Join the American Diabetes Association (ADA). You will receive a monthly subscription to *Diabetes Forecast*, the most informative journal written for people with diabetes and their family. Every issue focuses on a famous person living with diabetes and how he or she deals with it.

I have been inspired by many people who live with type 1 diabetes. One of these role models whose career I followed in the early days after my diagnosis was Mary Tyler Moore, a very funny and dynamic actress on several sitcoms in the 1970s and 1980s. I enjoyed her shows even before I was diagnosed with diabetes. Cathy Feste, the author of *The Physician Within, Tips & Tales From 50 Years With Diabetes*, and *365 Daily Meditations for People With Diabetes*, spoke at a seminar on living with diabetes and wrote letters to members of the ADA. In one of these letters she wrote that she was a parent chaperone for her son's trip, which included rafting down a turbulent river. One of the boys in the group said he could not go because he had diabetes. That surprised her, because she never thought of her diabetes as a reason not to go. She got her positive attitude from her mother, who announced to her, at age ten, that because of her health issue the entire family would lead a very healthy lifestyle. At the time, Cathy was hospitalized and had just been diagnosed with type 1 diabetes. What a wise mother she had! I also met a man who had type 1 diabetes for seventy years. He had been diagnosed with diabetes at the age of twelve and was one of the first children given dog insulin in the 1920s. He had no complications and was healthy enough to travel from the Midwest to attend a meeting sponsored by the ADA in Virginia. One of my neighbors also provided me with inspiration. She was two when she was diagnosed and had lived through all of the chaos of the rebellious teenage years and the wild partying of her college days. Despite all of this she had no damaging long-term complications and, at thirty-eight, is living a very active life with her husband and daughter. People such as these keep me motivated and help me to get back on track when I don't pay attention to what I am doing.

What Nurses Know...

You may require some sort of "cheering section" to handle making large changes in your life. Without enough encouragement, sometimes we simply may not be able to motivate ourselves enough from within.

Set a start date to get motivated soon, like tomorrow or the next day. To keep yourself accountable, write it on your calendar with a big star. Post it on your bathroom mirror, on your computer, your lunch bag, your briefcase, and so on. Make it happen whether or not you are ready. Make a plan, a grocery list, plan an activity with or without an exercise buddy, and then just do it! You can modify the plan as you learn more about diabetes and your body. It is very important that you start something different NOW!

If you are still wondering how to get motivated, look at the big picture. Decide what you really want out of life, then make it happen. Find a way to do it despite the fact that you have diabetes—maybe *because* you have diabetes. Having diabetes should never

What Nurses Know...

Make small monthly goals that are reasonably obtained within the given time span. Crossing things off your list is the ultimate motivator!

be an excuse for not accomplishing something. What do you find worthwhile? What turns you on? How do you want to live the rest of your life? This may require a lot of soul searching, especially if you are less driven than I am, which is not a bad thing. Believe me, being a perfectionist has its downside, especially when it come to diabetes control. For you this diagnosis may give direction to your life, a purpose for living life to the fullest, to experiment with food, exercise, stress management, and so on, and see how they relate to your blood glucose levels. Before I was diagnosed with diabetes, I would never have spent my time developing low-carb recipes.

Use your imagination. Picture yourself in a dangerous situation in which you need to run away to be safe, or a happy situation in which your kids or grandkids want you to actively play with them. Could you? If not, now is the time to work on getting the stamina to do it. Every time you want to quit, think of your imaginary situation and keep at it.

One more motivating point is that if you cannot or will not control your blood sugars, you will be constantly at risk for hyper- or hypoglycemia and you should not be driving a car. Remember that you may feel fine until your blood sugar is over 250 mg/dl or under 60 mg/dl, which encompasses a large area of unknown. Hyperglycemia will make you sleepy and blur your vision. Hypoglycemia will cause you to be confused and unable to process information, slow your reflexes, also blur your vision, and may cause a coma or a seizure. For twenty years, I had a forty-minute commute to and from work, and I always tested my blood sugar before I started my car. Most of the time it was OK, but the fear of causing an accident and injuring myself and others kept me from omitting this task. If my blood sugar was high, I gave myself insulin, and if it was low I always had glucose tablets in my purse. Waiting fifteen minutes for whatever treatment I needed to take effect delayed my return home, so I diligently worked at making that unnecessary. The more you monitor your blood sugar, aim for tight control, and follow a healthy lifestyle, the less likely you will be an accident waiting to happen.

I love slogans, as you have probably guessed, and there is one I have paraphrased that has inspired me over the years: "It is better to light one candle (try something new) than to curse the darkness (your diabetes)." Albert Einstein once defined insanity as "doing something over and over again expecting a different result." If your life, health, and diabetes are out of control, make a new plan. Make it realistic and doable. Make it specific, and make yourself accountable. Put it on your calendar, PDA, or iPhone. And there should be no ifs, ands, or buts—period!

Value the *journey* rather than the destination. Look forward to learning more about diabetes; experimenting with new technologies, new foods, new ways of being active; and understanding how this affects your diabetes, your body, and your life. Work at putting it all together. The destination may or may not be "perfect" blood sugar levels. It may be living a healthy lifestyle, enjoying family and friends, being independent, and so on. There will still be disappointments, discouraging blood sugars, perhaps the development of a complication or two, or times when you need help from a healthcare professional or a family member or friend. Use these occasions as opportunities to learn and grow. You may be knocked down, but don't let yourself be out for the count. Pick yourself up and move on. Successful people in any endeavor are flexible, adaptable, resilient, and self-forgiving. They are *not* perfect. Only you have control over what you do about anything that happens, so enjoy the ride, bumps, curves, detours and all.

Regardless of whether or not you can see yourself as motivated enough to do what you know you need to do, you will be correct every time. If you cannot imagine yourself eating a healthy diet, exercising regularly, and testing your blood sugar levels even when they are discouraging, it won't happen. If you think you can do it, you will do it. Remember the children's book about the *Little Engine That Could.* I think I can, I think I can!

Where there's a will, there's a way. You can do it. If you can do it, your family can do it. If your family as a whole can do it, your kids can do it. If your children can do it, their friends can do it, and so on. WOW! And it all started with you. Impressive!

Glossary

Acanthosis nigricans is a condition characterized by discolored patches in the skin folds of the armpits, neck, or groin, ranging from tan to dark brown. Acanthosis nigricans is associated with hyperinsulinemia (a higher-than-normal level of insulin in the blood), which results from obesity-related insulin resistance.

ACE inhibitor or angiotensin converting enzyme inhibitor is an antihypertensive which prevents an enzyme from causing the conversion of angiotensinogen to angiotensin constricting blood vessels and thus raising blood pressure.

Adhesion is a band of scar-like tissue that forms between two surfaces inside the body and causes them to stick together. The causes include surgery, trauma. and inflammation. This can happen anywhere in the body such as in joints and inside the abdomen or pelvis.

Aerobic exercise is any physical exercise that requires additional effort by the heart and lungs to meet increased demand by the skeletal muscles for oxygen resulting in incresed heart and lung efficiency.

Alpha cells are cells in the Islets of Langerhans of the pancreas that produce glucagon which causes the liver to release stored glucose in the form of glycogen.

Alpha-glucosidase inhibitors work in the small intestine to delay and/or block the digestion of carbohydrates (starches and sucrose) and decrease the peak after meal glucose levels allowing insulin production to better match glucose absorption. Examples include Precose and Glyset.

Amsler Grid is a series of vertical and horizontal lines with a dot in the middle. The Amsler Grid may be used on a daily basis, testing each eye separately. In this way, someone with macular degeneration will become familiar with their own pattern of distortion. Any new waviness should be reported to their doctor. This may be a sign of active "wet" macular degeneration.

Amylin is a hormone produced by the beta cells of the pancreas as is insulin. It is secreted in response to eating and helps to reduce post meal glucagon levels thus lowering blood glucose. Symlin is a synthetic amylin analog.

Anaerobic exercise is exertion of muscles without the need to take in more oxygen.

Antihypertensives are drugs that lower blood pressure.

Antihyperlipademics are drugs that lower cholesterol.

ARB stands for angiotensin receptor blocker. It is a type of antihypertensive that prevents blood pressure from going up by blocking the receptors for angiotensin, a powerful substance which makes the blood vessels contract causing blood pressure to rise.

Arrhythmia is any deviation from the normal pattern of the heartbeat or an irregular beat.

Atherosclerosis occurs when fatty deposits stick to the inner layers of the walls of large and medium arteries.

Autonomic neuropathy is the inflammation or degeneration of nerves in the autonomic nervous system caused by hyperglycemia. Neurogenic bladder, gastroporesis, and erectile dysfunction are examples.

Basal metabolic rate (BMR) is the amount of energy used by a fasting, resting person to maintain vital functions.

Beta blockers are antihypertensives that block Beta receptors on blood vessels so stress hormones can not cause them to constrict. They also prevent the increase in heart rate.

Beta cells of the islets of Langerhans produce insulin in response to a rise in blood glucose.

Biguanides are antidiabetic drugs that act primarily to decrease the liver's inappropriate release of glycogen into the blood, thus increasing blood sugar. It also improves tissue insulin sensitivity, both problems in type 2 diabetes. Glucophage, Glumetza, and Fortamet are examples.

Body mass index (BMI) is a calculation of body fatness based on the relationship between a person's height and weight. It is calculated by using body weight in kilograms divided by height in meters squared.

Calcium channel blockers (CCBs) slow the movement of calcium into the cells of the heart and blood vessel walls, which makes it easier for the heart to pump and widens blood vessels.

Carb counting is a method of keeping track of the number of grams of carbohydrates for weight loss and blood sugar control. Foods high in dietary carbohydrates include sugar, starchy foods like potatoes and pasta, and grain-based foods like breads and cereals. Carbohydrates can also be found in dairy products and fruits and starchy vegetables, as well as many beverages.

Cardiovascular disease refers to conditions or diseases of the heart and blood vessels in general, including coronary artery disease, angina, congestive heart failure, and high blood pressure, and stroke.

Carotid artery is the main artery carrying oxygenated blood from from the heart to the brain. There is one on each side of the neck.

Carotid endarterectomy is a surgical procedure used to prevent stroke, by correcting the stenosis (narrowing) in the common carotid artery. Endarterectomy is the removal of material on the inside (end-) of an artery.

Carotinoids are precursors to vitamin A found in yellow and orange vegetables.

Carpal tunnel syndrome is a median nerve entrapment, often caused by repetitive motion, such typing or painting, that irritates the tendons around the median nerve at the wrist. This causes swelling, which makes the bony tunnel space narrower and compresses the nerve.

Cerebral arteries are the arteries in the brain carrying oxygenated blood to the cells of the brain.

Charcot's joint or neuropathic osteoarthropathy, also known as Charcot arthropathy (often "Charcot foot"), refers to progressive degeneration of a weight bearing joint, a process marked by bony destruction, bone resorption, and eventual deformity.

Cholesterol is a sterol lipid (fat) synthesized by the liver and transported in the bloodstream to the membranes of all animal cells; it plays a central role in many biochemical processes and, as a lipoprotein that coats the walls of blood vessels, is associated with cardiovascular disease. Cholesterol can also be found in many animal food sources.

Congenial anomalies are birth defects.

Congestive heart failure is a condition caused by the inadequacy of the heart so that as a pump it fails to maintain the circulation of blood by pumping it forward, with the result that congestion and edema develop in the tissues first in the lungs and then in the rest of the body.

Continuous glucose monitoring systems (CGMS) are devices that test blood glucose levels every 5 minutes or so depending on the system. This continues for 72 hours or more before the site must be changed and wirelessly transmits the information to a receiver (cell phone size) or an insulin pump which displays the results.

Continuous Positive Airway Pressure (CPAP) machine is a small apparatus that pressurizes air and blows it through a hose attached to a mask worn at night to keep the airway open and prevent apnic spells.

Coronary artery disease (CAD) is a narrowing or blockage of the arteries and vessels that provide oxygen and nutrients to the heart muscle.

Crohn's Disease A chronic inflammatory disease, primarily involving the small and large intestine, but that can affect other parts of the digestive system as well.

CT scan or computed tomography scan (also known as a CAT scan) is a computerized x-ray procedure. A CT scan produces cross-sectional images of the body. The images are far more detailed than x-ray films, and can reveal disease or abnormalities in tissue and bone. The procedure is usually noninvasive and brief.

DASH diet or Dietary Alternative to Stop Hypertension includes fresh fruit, vegetables, and whole grain products. It is a diet high in potassium and low in sodium.

Dermopathy also called shin spots is a skin condition that develops as a result of changes to the blood vessels that supply the skin as a result of hyperglycemia. Dermopathy appears as a shiny round or oval lesion of thin skin over the front lower parts of the lower legs. The patches do not hurt, although rarely they can be itchy or cause burning. Medical treatment generally is not necessary.

Diabetes self-management is a pro-active way to look at client-controlled management of a complex disease. It involves the client's willingness to learn how to control the disease, take the steps to actively participate in the treatment, seek help when needed, and is willing to self-tailor this treatment based on knowledge of his/her own body.

Diabetic ketoacidosis (DKA) is a condition that occurs when the body can not burn glucose for energy since there is insufficient insulin to move it into cells. The body then burns fat and the byproduct of this burning creates fatty acids and ketones.

Dietary Guidelines for Americans The Dietary Guidelines are jointly issued and updated every 5 years by the U.S. Departments of Agriculture (USDA) and Health and Human Services (HHS). They provide authoritative advice for people two years and older about how good dietary habits can promote health and reduce risk for major chronic diseases.

DPP-4 inhibitor class of medications (like Januvia and Onglyxa) helps the body lower too-high blood glucose levels in people with type 2 diabetes by increased incretin levels (GLP-1 and GIP), which inhibit glucagon release, the effect of which, in turn, decreases blood glucose, but, more significantly, increases insulin secretion and slows gastric emptying.

Diuretics make kidneys excrete more water in the urine thus lowering blood pressure.

Endocrinologist is a physician who specializes in the diagnosis and treatment of conditions affecting the endocrine system including the thyroid and the pancreas.

Fat-soluble vitamins are vitamins that dissolve in dietary and body fat (vitamins A, D, E, and K). They are metabolized and absorbed only in the presence of dietary fat. Because excess fat-soluble vitamins may be stored in the body fat, several weeks' supply may be consumed in a single dose or meal.

Fetal demise is death of the fetus during pregnancy.

Fetal surveillance is an indirect way to measure fetal well-being and the adequacy of fetal oxygenation and includes periodic ultrasound, fetal monitoring, fetal movement assessment, periodic fetal heart rate, continuous electronic fetal heart rate monitoring, fetal amniotic fluid analysis, and more.

Frozen shoulder or adhesive capsulitis is a painful restriction of shoulder movement.

Gestation is another word for pregnancy.

Gestational age is how many weeks old a fetus is.

Gestational diabetes mellitus (GDM) is diabetes that occurs only during pregnancy.

Gingivitis is the inflammation of gums in the mouth. Gums become red, swollen, and often bleed.

Glomerulus is a capillary tuft in the kidney that performs the first step in filtering blood to form urine.

Glucose is a simple sugar. Cells use it as a source of energy. Glucose is one of the main products of photosynthesis. Starch and cellulose are polymers derived from the dehydration of glucose.

Glucose challenge test measures the amount of glucose (sugar) in the blood stream after the woman is "challenged" with a 50 gram glucose solution. It determines whether she can produce enough insulin in one hour to keep blood sugar levels from rising. This test is given between 24 and 28 weeks of pregnancy to screen for gestational diabetes.

Glucose tolerance test is the administration of a premeasured amount of glucose drink (usually 75 to 100 grams) to determine how quickly it is cleared from the blood and homeostasis is maintained. The test is usually used to test for diabetes, insulin resistance, and sometimes reactive hypoglycemia.

Glycogen in the glucose that is stored in the liver and skeletal muscles for later use.

Glycosuria or glucosuria is a condition that exists when glucose is found in urine.

Hemodialysis is a method for removing waste products such as creatinine and urea, as well as free water from the blood when the kidneys are in renal failure.

Heart failure is a condition in which a problem with the structure or function of the heart impairs its ability to supply sufficient blood flow to meet the body's needs.

Hemoglobin A1c is a blood test that measures the average percentage of blood glucose over a 2-3 month period. It can be used to diagnose diabetes.

High-density lipoprotein (HDL) is a type of lipoprotein that consists of about 50% protein and 19% cholesterol. It protects against cardiovascular disease by removing cholesterol deposits from arteries or preventing their formation. It is also known as good cholesterol.

HLA markers or human leukocyte antigens are antigens associated with specific autoimmune diseases. Some HLA antigens offer protection against certain autoimmune diseases. We get these genetic markers from our biological parents.

Hydrogenated fat is unsaturated fat to which hydrogen has been added to make it more stable and solid at room temperature. Partially or completely hydrogenated oils both contain trans fat.

Hypercholesterolemia is another name for high cholesterol levels in the blood.

Hyperglycemia is another word for high blood sugar and is usually defined as 180 mg/dl or higher but symptoms may not start to become noticeable until blood glucose is over 250 mg/dl.

Hyperinsulinemia means a higher-than-normal level of insulin in the blood. This is common in overweight and obese individuals who are insulin resistant. They may or may not develop diabetes.

Hyperosmolar hyperglycemic nonketosic syndrome (HHNS) is a serious condition most frequently seen in older persons with type 2 diabetes caused by an illness or infection. Blood sugar level are usually over 600 mg/dl and there is severe dehydration from the kidneys' attempt to get rid of the glucose. There is enough insulin produced to use some of the sugar so fat is not burned for energy (nonketosis). Severe dehydration may lead to seizures, coma and eventually death.

Hyperthyroidism is an autoimmune disease caused by overactive tissue within the thyroid gland, resulting in overproduction and thus an excess of circulating free thyroid hormones: thyroxin (T4), triiodothyronine (T3), or both. Symptoms include nervousness, irritability, increased perspiration, a fast heart rate, hand tremors, anxiety, difficulty sleeping, thinning of the skin, fine brittle hair, and muscular weakness especially in the upper arms and thighs. Weight loss, sometimes significant, despite a good appetite may occur, as well as vomiting, and, for women, menstrual flow may lighten and menstrual periods may occur less often.Treatment includes medically obliterating the thyroid gland or surgically removing it.

Hypoglycemia is another word for low blood sugar, usually defined as lower than 70 mg/dl. Glucose levels of 40 and below constitute severe hypoglycemia, a life-threatening emergency.

Hypothyroidism is an autoimmune disease caused by decreased activity of the thyroid gland. Symptoms may include weight gain, sluggishness, dry skin, intolerance to cold, and slowing of bodily processes. Treatment includes prescribing oral dosages of the thyroid hormone.

Incretin mimetics is a synthetic version of the human incretin hormone GLP-1 (glucagon-like peptide-1) that is secreted in the small intestines, but it lasts longer. This drug classification includes Byetta (exenatide) and Victoza (liraglutide).

Insulin analogs are a man-made substances resembling insulin in which the molecular structure has been altered for a more desirable effect. Some insulin analogs are rapid acting (Humalog, NovoLog, Apidra) or long acting (Lantus, Levemir).

Insulin to carbohydrate ratios is the ratio between one unit of insulin and the specific number of grams of carbohydrates it will take care of, such as 1 unit to 10 grams of carbs.

Intermittent claudication is a pain in one or both legs that a person experiences when walking or exercising due to insufficient blood flow to bring enough oxygen to the active muscle. The pain is intermittent and goes away when the person rests.

Interstitial fluid is fluid between the cells of the body.

Ischemia is caused by inadequate blood supply to tissue from blocked blood vessels to the area.

Islets of Langerhans are irregular clusters of endocrine cells scattered throughout the tissue of the pancreas that secrete insulin and glucagon. They are named after Paul Langerhans, the German scientist who discovered them in 1869.

Ketonemia occurs when fat is burned for energy and the byproduct, ketones, build up in the blood.

Ketonuria is a condition in which ketones from fat metabolism are present in the urine.

Lactation is another word for the process of breastfeeding.

Large-for-gestational age means that a newborn is larger than the range of normal weight at that gestational age or greater that the 90th percentile for that gestational age. For example, a baby born at 40 weeks gestation should weight between 6.6 and 8.8 lbs.

Laser photocoagulation is the coagulation (clotting) of tissue using a laser which produces light in the visible green wavelength that is selectively absorbed by hemoglobin, the pigment in red blood cells. It is used to seal off bleeding blood vessels in the back of the eye.

Low-density lipoprotein (LDL) is a type of lipoprotein that transports cholesterol and triglycerides from the liver to peripheral tissues and blood vessels. Since higher levels of LDL particles promote health problems and cardiovascular disease, they are often called bad cholesterol.

Macrosomia leads to a large for gestational age (LGA) baby whose birth weight lies above the 90th percentile for that gestational age.

Macular degeneration is a medical condition that usually affects older adults that results in a loss of vision in the center of the visual field (the macula) because of damage to the retina. It occurs in "dry" and "wet" forms. It is a major cause of visual impairment in older adults (>50 years). Macular degeneration can make it difficult or impossible to read or recognize faces, although enough peripheral vision remains to allow other activities of daily life.

Magnetic resonance imaging (MRI) involves the use of nuclear magnetic resonance of protons to produce proton density images.

Meglitinide is a classification of drugs that make the pancreas produce more insulin in response to glucose. It works much faster than sulfonylureas and does not last as long. Prandin is the only example to date and should be taken right before a meal.

Metabolic syndrome is a condition that includes obesity, insulin resistance, diabetes or pre-diabetes, hypertension and high lipids.

Microalbuminuria is a small amounts of protein found in the urine. It is a highly sensitive indicator of glomerular disease and a sign that kidneys are not functioning properly.

Monounsaturated fat is a kind of fat in which one or more pairs of electrons in the atom making up the fat molecule form a bond with a pair of electrons from another atom (a double bond).

Monounsaturated fats contain one double bond and are found in peanuts, peanut butter, olives, and avocados. They are heart-healthy fats.

Necrobiosis lipoidica diabeticorum (NLD) is a condition thought to be caused by changes in the collagen and fat content underneath the skin. The overlaying skin area becomes thinned and reddened. Most lesions are found on the lower parts of the legs and can ulcerate if subjected to trauma. Sometimes, NLD is itchy and painful.

Nephrons are the working units of the kidney that remove waste and extra fluids from the blood. Each kidney is made of approximately 1 million nephrons.

Nephropathy is a serious kidney disease that can occur in people who have had diabetes for a long time, particularly if their diabetes has been poorly controlled.

Neuropathy refers to any disease or injury affecting nerves or nerve cells.

Noncompliance is the failure or refusal of a knowledgeable and financially able person to cooperate and carry out those activities that have been communicated to this person by healthcare practitioners as being appropriate to control the disease and therefore exerts his or her own control knowing that by doing so he or she is purposely shortening life expectancy.

Nonproliferative retinopathy is the initial stage in diabetic retinopathy. High levels of blood glucose cause damage to the blood vessels in the retina. The blood vessels leak fluid, which can collect and cause the retina to swell. This stage usually does not cause decrease in vision.

Normoglycemic means having a normal amount of glucose in the blood. Normal fasting blood sugar is 70 to 99 mg/dl.

Olestra or Olean is a fat substitute that adds no fat, calories, or cholesterol to products. It has been used in the preparation of traditionally high-fat foods such as potato chips, thereby lowering or eliminating their fat content.

Ophthalmologist is a medical doctor, who diagnoses and treats all diseases and disorders of the eye including surgical treatment. They can also prescribe glasses and contact lenses.

Optometrist is a doctor of optometry (OD), a primary healthcare professional for the eye. Optometrists examine, diagnose, treat, and manage diseases, injuries, and disorders of the eye. They prescribe glasses, contact lenses and low vision aids. Optometrist can not perform surgery.

Pancreatitis is an inflammation of the pancreas. It can be acute or chronic and can be caused by alcoholism, trauma, infection, and some drugs. It can be extremely painful and may require treatment with pancreatic digestive hormones as well as insulin as it heals.

Pedometer is a device worn on the belt usually on one side. It counts steps, can calculate miles walked and some may calculate pound lost, heart rate and other information based on parameters pre-programmed into it by user.

Periodontal disease is a set of inflammatory diseases affecting the tissues that surround and support the teeth. Periodontitis involves progressive loss of the alveolar bone around the teeth, and if left untreated, can lead to the loosening and subsequent loss of teeth.

Peripheral artery disease (PAD) includes all diseases caused by the obstruction of large arteries in the arms and legs.

Peripheral neuropathy is a condition of the nervous system that usually begins in the hands and/or feet with symptoms of numbness, tingling, burning and/or weakness. It can be caused by certain anticancer drugs and by hyperglycemia.

Peritoneal dialysis is a treatment for persons with severe chronic kidney failure. The process uses the peritoneum in the abdomen as a membrane across which fluids and dissolved substances (electrolytes, urea, glucose, albumin and other small molecules) are exchanged from the blood. Fluid is introduced through a permanent tube in the abdomen and flushed out either every night while the person sleeps (automatic peritoneal dialysis) or via regular exchanges throughout the day (continuous ambulatory peritoneal dialysis).

Peritonitis is an infection of the gut wall or peritoneum. It can be a complication of peritoneal dialysis or from a ruptured appendix or other causes of abdominal infection.

Pilates is an exercise system that is focused on building strength without bulk, improving flexibility and agility, and helping to prevent injury.

Placebo an inert compound or treatment that should have no effect. The **placebo effect** is when the client expects something to happen and it does, even though the client was not given the *real* medication or treatment.

Podiatrist is a Doctor of Podiatric Medicine (DPM), also known as a podiatric physician or surgeon who is qualified by their education and training to diagnose and treat conditions affecting the foot, ankle and related structures of the leg.

Polyunsaturated fat is a kind of fat in which one or more pairs of electrons in the atom making up the fat molecule form a bond with a pair of electrons from another atom (a double bond). Polyunsaturated fats contain two or more double bonds and are found in oils such as corn, sunflower, and soybean. They are heart-healthy fats.

Postprandial means after meals.

Preconception means prior to pregnancy and usually refers to pre-pregnancy health evaluation and care.

Prediabetes occurs when there is impaired fasting glucose, impaired glucose tolerance, a fasting glucose of 100 to 125 mg/dl or an A1c between 5.7 to 6.4%. Those with prediabetes have an increased risk of developing diabetes in the near future if weight loss and lifestyle changes are not instituted.

PreDx Diabetes Risk Score Test is a simple blood test that Tethys Bioscience says can identify persons with a high risk of developing type 2 diabetes within five years.

Pregestational means before pregnancy.

Pregnancy-induced hypertension (PIH) is hypertension after 20 weeks of pregnancy that is accompanied by proteinuria and edema above the waist. It is a dangerous condition of pregnancy that can develop over a number of weeks or it can have a sudden onset and end in convulsions. Older terms are pre-eclampsia (before a seizure) and eclampsia (seizure).

Prematurity means before 37 completed weeks or the 1st day of the 38th week.

Preprandial means before meals.

Proliferative retinopathy is the fourth stage of diabetic retinopathy, where signals sent by the retina for nourishment, trigger the growth of new blood vessels which are abnormal and fragile. They grow along the retina and the surface of the clear vitreous gel that fills the inside of the eye. They can bleed into the vitreous gel ans cause blurred vision or blindness if bleeding is extensive.

Proteinuria is a condition in which an excessive amount of protein is found in the urine.

Renal tubules are the microscopic chemical factories in the kidneys that manufacture urine from filtered blood, at the same time conserving essential nutrients and other substances required by the body like protein.

Retina is the light-sensitive lining of the back of the eye ball which transmits signals to the optic nerve which sends them to the brain for interpretation.

Retinopathy is a complication of diabetes that is caused by changes in the blood vessels of the retina. When blood vessels in the retina are damaged, they may leak blood and grow fragile, brush-like branches and scar tissue. This can blur or distort the vision images that the retina sends to the brain.

Rheumatoid arthritis (RA) is a chronic autoimmune disease with inflammation of the joints and marked deformities; something (possibly a virus) triggers an attack on the joint by the immune system, which releases cytokines that stimulate an inflammatory reaction that can lead to the destruction of all components of the joint.

Saturated fat is a type of fat that has been shown to increase the risk of heart disease. Found in animal foods such as butter, full fat dairy foods, and fatty meats, as well as many processed and take-out foods.

Scleroderma diabeticorum is a skin problem that affects people with type 2 diabetes, causing a thickening of the skin on the back of the neck and upper back.

Secretagogue medication are drugs that make the pancreas increase its production of insulin.

SGLT2 inhibitors work by inhibiting the SGLT2 molecule (sodium-glucose co-transporter) in the kidney tubules that cause reabsorption of sugar and sodium that otherwise would be excreted in the urine. The result is that more sugar and sodium are excreted resulting in lower blood sugar, weight loss and lower blood pressure. Dapgliflozin and canagliflozin are examples but no drugs in this class are yet on the market.

Standard of care is the treatment that another prudent healthcare professional, of similar backgrounds and training, would give to the same client. It is usually the recommended treatment option for this person for this problem.

Stent is a man-made 'tube' inserted into a natural passage/conduit in the body to prevent, or counteract, a disease-induced, localized flow constriction. It is used as part of an angioplasty procedure to correct a blockage in a coronary or peripheral artery such as in the leg.

Sugar alcohols are food additives that are used as sweeteners and texturizing agents in foods. The limited absorption and metabolism of sugar alcohols are important factors in their use in dietetic foods. The list includes mannitol, sorbitol, xylitol, maltitol and other *itol* sweeteners. They do contribute to blood sugar but are slowly absorbed. They also stimulate the bowels and even a listed serving size may cause cramps and diarrhea in some people.

Sulfonylureas are a group of hypoglycemic drugs that act on the beta cells of the pancreas to increase the secretion of insulin.

Systemic lupus erythematosis (SLE) is a chronic autoimmune connective tissue disease that can affect any part of the body. As occurs in other autoimmune diseases, the immune system attacks the body's cells and tissue, resulting in inflammation and tissue damage.

Tai Chi is a Chinese system of slow meditative physical exercise designed for relaxation, balance, and health.

Thiazolidinedione (TZD) is a class of drugs (such as pioglitazone and rosiglitazone) that are thiazolidine derivatives used to reduce insulin resistance in the treatment of type 2 diabetes.

Trans fat is a type of unsaturated fat with trans-isomer fatty acid(s), usually made by food manufacturers by partially hydrogenating mono or polyunsaturated oils so that foods last longer on shelves or in cans. Eating trans fats increases the risk of some illnesses, such as heart disease.

Transient ischemic attacks (TIA) is a risk factor for stroke, TIAs are caused by temporary interruptions to the blood supply of the brain. TIA symptoms are similar to stroke symptoms but disappear within a few minutes.

Trigger finger, trigger thumb, or trigger digit, is a common disorder of later adulthood characterized by catching, snapping or locking of the involved finger flexor tendon, associated with dysfunction and pain. It can be corrected with outpatient surgery or eased with massage and stretching exercises.

Triglycerides is a common blood fat that triggers the liver to create more cholesterol. If blood glucose is high, triglycerides are usually high. Elevated triglycerides can also be due to overweight/obesity, physical inactivity, cigarette smoking, excess alcohol consumption and a diet very high in carbohydrates (60 percent of total calories or more).

Type 1 diabetes mellitus is a form of diabetes mellitus that results from autoimmune destruction of insulin-producing beta cells of the pancreas. The subsequent lack of insulin leads to increased blood and urine glucose.

Type 2 diabetes mellitus is a disorder that is characterized by high blood glucose in the context of insulin resistance and relative insulin deficiency.

Valsalva maneuver is performed by forcible exhalation against a closed airway, usually done by closing one's mouth as in pushing down to have a stool.

Vitrectomy is a surgical procedure that removes the vitreous gel from the back of the eye and replace it with saline solution. It is usually an outpatient procedure done under local anesthesia.

Water-soluble vitamins are not stored in the body and must be replenished on a daily basis. Water-soluble vitamins include the B complex of vitamins (thiamin, riboflavin, niacin, pyridoxine, biotin, folic acid, B6 and B12) and vitamin C.

Xerostomia means dry mouth.

Yoga is a healing system of theory and practice. It is a combination of breathing exercises, physical postures, and meditation that has been practiced for more than 5,000 years.

Resources

The following is a list of diabetes organizations and diabetes professionals.

American Association of Diabetes Educators
100 West Monroe, 4th Floor
Chicago, IL 60603-1901
Phone: 800-338-3633 for names of diabetes educators
312-424-2426 to order publications
www.aadenet.org

American Association of Kidney Patients
3505 East Frontage Rd., Suite 315
Tampa, FL 33607
Phone: 800-749-2257
E-mail: info@aakp.org
www.aakp.org

American Diabetes Association

1701 North Beauregard St.
Alexandria, VA 22311
Phone: 703-549-1500
800-ADA-ORDER to order publications toll free
800-DIABETES (800-342-2383) for
diabetes information
www.diabetes.org

American Dietetic Association

National Center for Nutrition and Dietetics
216 West Jackson Blvd., Suite 800
Chicago, IL 60606-6995
Phone: 800-366-1655 Consumer Nutrition Hotline (Spanish
   speaker available)
800-745-0775
www.eatright.org

American Heart Association National Center

7272 Greenville Ave.
Dallas, TX 75231
Phone: 214-373-6300
www.heart.org/heartorg

American Kidney Fund

6110 Executive Blvd., Suite 1010
Rockville, MD 20852
Phone: 800-638-8299 or 301-881-3052
E-mail: helpline@kidneyfund.org
www.kidneyfund.org

American Pain Foundation

201 North Charles St., Suite 710
Bethesda, MD 21201-4111
Phone: 888-615-7246 or 410-385-1832
www.painfoundation.org

American Podiatric Medical Association
9312 Old Georgetown Rd.
Bethesda, MD 20814-1621
Phone: 800-FOOTCARE (366-8227) or 301-581-9200
www.apma.org

American Psychological Association 750 First St., NE,
Washington, DC 20002-4242 Phone: 800-374-2723
www.apa.org/, http://locator.apa.org

To find a therapist versed in cognitive behavior therapy in your
state, go to www.psychologyinfo.com/directory/state-links.html

American Urological Association Foundation
1000 Corporate Blvd.
Linthicum, MD 21090
Phone: 866-746-4282 or 410-689-3700
www.auafoundation.org, www.urologyhealth.org

Diabetes Exercise and Sports Association
310 West Liberty, Suite 604
Louisville, KY 40202
Phone: 800-898-4322
Fax: 502-581-0206
www.diabetes-exercise.org

Juvenile Diabetes Research Foundation International
26 Broadway
New York, NY 10004
Phone: 800-533-CURE (800-533-2873)
Fax: 212-785-9595
www.jdrf.org

Life Options Rehabilitation Program
c/o Medical Education Institute, Inc.
414 D'Onofrio Dr., Suite 200
Madison, WI 53719
Phone: 800-468-7777 or 608-232-2333

E-mail: lifeoptions@meiresearch.org
www.lifeoptions.org, www.kidneyschool.org

Lower Extremity Amputation Prevention Program
Health Resources and Services Administration
5600 Fishers Ln.
Rockville, MD 20857
Phone: 888-ASK-HRSA (888-275-4772)
www.hrsa.gov/leap

National Diabetes Information Clearinghouse
1 Information Way
Bethesda, MD 20892-3560
Phone: 301-654-3327 or 800-860-8747
www.diabetes.niddk.nih.gov

National Kidney Foundation, Inc.
30 East 33rd St.
New York, NY 10016
Phone: 800-622-9010 or 212-889-2210
www.kidney.org

The Neuropathy Associations, Inc.
60 E. 42nd St., Suite 942
New York, NY 10165-0999
Phone: 800-247-6968
www.neuropathy.org

Periodicals

The following journals and magazines deal with diabetes and
self-care management:

Diabetes Forecast, http://forecast.diabetes.org
Diabetes Self-Management, www.diabetesselfmanagement.com
Diabetic Living, www.diabeticlivingonline.com
Diabetic Cooking, www.diabeticcooking.com

Diabetes Health, www.diabeteshealth.com
Eating Well, www.eatingwell.com
Insulin, www.insulinjournal.com

Organizations that have information about diabetes and other health issues:

Federal Government Organizations

Centers for Disease Control and Prevention
1600 Clifton Rd.
Atlanta, GA 30333
800-CDC-INFO (800-232-4636) or 770-488-5000
www.cdc.gov/diabetes

Health Resources and Services Administration
5600 Fishers Ln.
Rockville, MD 20857
http://www.hrsa.gov

Indian Health Service
Diabetes Program
5300 Homestead Rd. NE
Albuquerque, NM 87110
505-248-4182
www.ihs.gov/medicalprograms/diabetes/index.asp

National Diabetes Education Program
One Diabetes Way
Bethesda, MD 20814-9692
Phone: 800-438-5383
http://ndep.nih.gov

National Institute of Diabetes and Digestive and Kidney Diseases
1 Information Way
Bethesda, MD 20892-3560
Phone: 800-GET LEVEL (800-438-5383) or 301-654-3327
www.niddk.nih.gov

National Diabetes Information Clearinghouse
1 Information Way
Bethesda, MD 20892-3560
Phone: 301-654-3327
Fax: 301-907-8906
diabetes.nddk.nih.gov/index.htm

National Eye Institute
Building 31, Room 6A32
31 Center Dr., MSC 2510
Bethesda, MD 20892-2510
Phone: 301-496-5248 or 800-869-2020 (to order materials)
Fax: 301-402-1065
www.nei.nih.gov

Office of Minority Health Resource Center
U.S. Department of Health and Human Services
P.O. Box 37337
Washington, DC 20013-7337
Phone: 800-444-MHRC (800-444-6472)
www.omhrc.gov

U.S. Department of Veterans Affairs
810 Vermont Ave., NW
Washington, DC 20420
www.va.gov/diabetes

Nonfederal Government Organizations

American Optometric Association
1505 Prince St.
Alexandria, VA 22314
Phone: 800-262-3947 or 703-739-9200
www.aoanet.org

American Podiatric Medical Association
9312 Old Georgetown Rd.

Bethesda, MD 20814
Phone: 301-571-9200 or 800-ASK-APMA (800-275-2762)
Fax: 301-530-2752
www.apma.org

Medical Eye Care for the Nation's Disadvantaged Senior Citizens

The Foundation of the American Academy of Ophthalmology
P.O. Box 429098
San Francisco, CA 94142-9098
Phone: 800-222-EYES (800-222-3937)
www.faao.org

Information on **living wills an advance directives** for each state:

National Hospices and Palliative Care Organization

Caring Connections
http://caringinfo.org

Equipment companies for current and future meters and other paraphernalia:

Meter Companies

Abbott Diabetes Care (formerly Therasense)

Phone: 888-522-5226, 800-527-3339
www.aboottdiabetescare.com
Meters: FreeStyle Lite, FreeStyle Freedom Lite, Precision Xtra

Accu-Chek

Phone: 800-858-8072
www.accu-chek.com/us
Meters: Aviva, Compact Plus, Active, Advantage

AgaMatrix, Inc.

Phone: 603-328-6000, 866-906-4197
www.wavesense.info
Meters: WaveSense Jazz, WaveSense KeyNote, WaveSense KeyNote Pro, WaveSense Presto, WaveSense Presto Pro

Arkray USA (formerly Hypoguard)
Phone: 800-818-8877
www.arkrayusa.com
Meters: Assure Platinum, Assure Pro, Assure 4
www.glucocarduse.com
Meters: Glucocard 01, Glucocard 01-Mini, Glucocard X-Meter,
  Glucocard Vital

Bayer
Phone: 800-348-8100
www.bayerdiabetes.com; www.simplewins.com
Meters: Breeze2, Contour, Contour TS A1C Now

Bionime USA
Phone: 888-481-8485
www.bionimeusa.com
Meters: Rightest GM100, Rigthest GM300

Diabetic Supply of Suncoast
Phone: 866-373-2824
www.pharmasupply.com
Meters: Advocate, Advocate Duo, Advocate Redi-Code

Diagnostic Devices
Phone: 800-243-2636
www.prodigymeter.com
Meters: Prodigy Autocode, Prodigy Pocket, Prodigy Voice

Fora Care
Phone: 866-469-2632
www.foracare.com/usa
Meters: Fora G20, Fora G90, Fora V10, Fora V12, Fora V20,
  Fora V22

Home Diagnostics
Phone: 800-342-7226, Ext. 3300
www.homediagnostics.com
Meters: Sidekick, True2Go, Trueresult, Truetrack

Infopia
Phone: 888-446-3246
www.infopiausa.com
Meters: Eclipse, Element, Envision, Evolution, GlucoLab

LifeScan
Phone: 800-227-8862
www.lifescan.com
Meters: One Touch UltraSmart, UltraMini, UltraMini2,
   UltraLink, Ulta2

Nova Biomedical
Phone: 800-681-7390
www.novacares.com
Meters: Nova Max, Nova Max Link

U.S. Diagnostics
Phone: 866-216-5308
www.usdiagnostics.net
Meters: Acura, EasyGluco, Infinity, Maxima

WalMart
Phone: 800-631-0076
www.relion.com/diabetes
Meters: ReliOn Micro, ReliOn Ultima

Insulin Pump Companies

Abbott Labs
Phone: 888-522-5226
www.abbottdiabetescare.com
Maker of FreeStyle Navigator
www.freestylenavigator.com

Animas
Phone: 877-937-7867
www.animascorp.com
Maker of the OneTouch Ping and 2020, IRI250, IR 1000
www.animas.com/Request-ping-pump-info

Disetronic

Phone: 800-280-7801

www.disetronic-usa.com

Makers of the Accu-Chek Spirit insulin pump

Insulet

Phone: 781-457-5000

www.myomnipod.com/about-omnipod/omnipod-CGM

Makers of the Omnipod Insulin pump

Metronic/MiniMed

Phone: 800-646-4633

www.minimed.com

Makers of the Paradigm 522/722 and Revel insulin pumps

Sooil Development Co. Ltd.

Phone: 858-404-0659

http//sooil.en.ec21.com/index.jsp

Makers of the Dana Diabecare II insulin pump

Tandem Diabetes Care

Phone: 858-366-6900

www.tandemdiabetes.com

Maker of t:slim insulin pump. Not available in the United States as of September 2010.

Continuous Monitor Companies

Abbott Diabetes

Phone: 866-597-5520

www.freestylenavigator.com

Makers of the Freestyle Navigator

Dexcom

Phone: 877-339-2664

www.dexcom.com

Maker of the Seven Plus System

Metronic/Minimed

Phone: 866-948-6633

www.minimed.com

Makers of the Paradigm Real Time System.

On-Line Resources

Cellnovo

www.cellnovo.com/#/products

dLife.com

www.dlife.com

iTunes

www.itunes.apple.com/us/app/diabetes-companion/
id360403719?mt=8

Drug Companies

Amylin Pharmaceuticals Inc.

Phone: 858-552-2200

Makers of Noninsulin injections

Symlin (pramlintide)

www.symlin.com

SymlinPen

www.symlin.com/132-using-the-symline-pen.aspx

Byetta (exenatide)

www.byetta.com/Pages/index.aspx

Bayer Pharmaceuticals Corp.

Makers of Precose (acarbose)

www.rxlist.com/precose-drug-patient.htm

Bristol-Myers Squibb Company

Makers of:

Glucophage (metformin) and Glucophage XR (metformin ER)

www.bms.com/ourcompany/Pages/uswebsites.aspx

Glucovance (metformin and glyburide)
www.rxlist.com/glucovance-drug-patient.htm
Metaglip (metformin and glipizide)
www.rxlist.com/metaglip-drug-patient.htm
Onglyza (saxagliptin)
www.onglyza.com/about/managing.aspx

DepoMed Inc.

Makers of Glumetza (metformin extended release)
www.depomedinc.com/view.cfm/1286/ourproducts

Eli Lilly & Company

Phone: 317-276-9624
Makers of:
Glucagon, Humulin R, N, Humulin 70/30, Humulin 50/50 vials
Humulin R, N, an d70/30 disposable, prefilled pens www.lillydi
  abetes.com/index.jsp
Humalog, Humalog 75/25 www.lillydiabetes.com/product/huma
  log.jsp?reNavId=5.1
Humalog KwikPen and Humalog 75/25 Prefilled Pen www.inside
  humalog.com/hcp/humalog_insulin_hcp.jsp

GlaxoSmithKline

Phone: 888-825-5249
Makers of:
Avandia (rosiglitazone)
www.avandia.com/
Avandamet (metformin and rosiglitazone) www.avandia.com/
  about_avandamet/avandmet.html
Avandaryl (rosiglitazone and glimepiride) www.rxlist.com/
  avandaryl-drug-patient.htm

Merck & Co. Inc.

Makers of:
Januvia (sitagliptin) www.januvia.com/sitagliptin/januvia/con-
sumer/index.jsp

Janumet (metformin and sitagliptin) www.janumet.com/sita
gliptin_metformin_HCl/janumet/consumer/medication_
guide/index.jsp

Novartis Pharmaceuticals USA

Phone: 888-669-6682

Makers of Starlix (netaglinide) www.pharma.us.novartis.com/
products/name/starlix.jsp

Novo Nordisk

800-727-6500

Makers of:

Prandin (repaglinide)

www.prandin.com

PrandiMet (metformin and Repaglinide)

www.rxlist.com/prandiment-drug-patient.htm

Novolin R, N vials and Novolin R, N and 70/30 Penfill

www.insulindevice.com/novopen/faq.asp

NovoLog and NovoLog 70/30

www.novolog.com, www.novologmix70-30.com

NovoLog Flexpen

www.novolog.com/devices-flexpen.asp?s=ds&h=60

Levemir and Levemir Flexpen

www.levemir-us.com

Victoza (liraglutide)

www.victoza.com

Glucagon

Pfizer Inc.

Phone: 212-733-2323

www.pfizer.com/products

Makers of: Diabenese, Glipiside, Glucotrol (glipizide) and
Glucatrol XL (glipizide ER), Glynase Pres tabs (micronized gly
buride), Glyset (miglitol), , Micronase (glyburide)

www.rxlist.com/glyset-drug-patient.htm

Ranboxy Pharmaceuticals
Makers of: Riomet (metformin oral solution)
www.riomet.com

Shionogi Pharma, Inc.
Makers of: Fortamet (metformin
extended release)
www.rxlist.com/fortament-drug-patient.htm

Sanofi-Aventis US
Phone: 800-633-1610
Makers of:
Diabeta (glyburdie)
www.sanofi-aventis.us/live/us/en/index.jsp
Amaryl (glimepiride)
www.sanofi-aventis.us/live/en/index.jsp
Apidra (glulisine insulin)
www.apidra.com/
Apidra SoloSTAR Pen Lantus (glargine insulin) and Lantus
   SoloSTAR Pen www.lantus.com/consumer/index.do

Takeda Pharmaceuticals
Makers of:
Actos (pioglitizone)
www.rxlist.com/actos-drug-patient.htm
Actoplus Met (metformin and pioglitazone)
www.rxlist.com/actoplus-met-drug-patient.htm
Duetact (pioglitazone and glimepiride)
www.actos.com/duetact/home.aspx

Nutrition

The following information relates to some of the Web sites listed
in Chapter 2:

Sugar-Free Syrups and Flavorings
Atkins Nutritionals, Inc.

Hauppauge, NY 11788
Phone: 800-6-ATKINS (800-628-5467)
www.lowcarb.ca/store/sauce.html

R. Torre & Co (maker of Torani Syrups)
So. San Francisco, CA 94080
www.torani.com

DaVinci Gourmet, Ltd.
Seattle, WA 98108
Phone: 800-640-6779
www.davincigourmet.com

Baja Bob's Sugar Free Cocktail Mixers
1465 Encinitas Blvd.
Encinitas, CA 92024
Phone: 888-569-2272, 760-634-5316
www.BajaBob.com

Low-Carb Pasta

Dakota Growers Pasta Company
One Past Ave.
Carrington, ND 58421
Phone: 800-250-1917
www.dreamfieldsfoods.com

Strumba Media LLC
8605 Santa Monica Blvd., Suite 6920
West Hollywood, CA 90065
Phone: 800-948-4205
www.miraclenoodle.com

Salt Substitutes

Mrs. Dash blend of herb and spices and marinades
Phone: 800-622-DASH
www.mrsdash.com

Morton's Lite Salt
Morton International, Inc

Chicago, IL 60606-1743 www.mortonsalt.com/products/food-salts/lite_salt.htm

DASH Diet (Dietary Approach to Stop Hypertension) http://dashdiet.org

References

Chapter 1

American Diabetes Association. (n.d.). *The genetics of diabetes.* http://www.diabetes.org/diabetes-basics/genetics-of-diabetes.html (accessed January 25, 2010).

American Diabetes Association. (2010). Standards of medical care in diabetes–2010. *Diabetes Care* 33:S11–S61.

Centers for Disease Control and Prevention. (2008). *National diabetes fact sheet, 2007.* http://www.cdc.gov/diabetes (accessed February 15, 2010).

Collazo-Clavell, M. (2009). *Mayo Clinic: The essential diabetes book.* New York: Time, Inc.

Mertig, R. G. (2007). *Nurses' guide to teaching diabetes self-management.* New York: Springer Publishing Company, LLC.

Rubin, A. L. (2008a). *Diabetes for dummies.* 3rd ed. Hoboken, NJ: Wiley.

Rubin, A. L. (2008b). *Type 1 diabetes for dummies.* Hoboken, NJ: Wiley.

Saudek, C. D., and Margolis, S. (2010). *Johns Hopkins white papers: Diabetes.* New York: MediZine LLC.

Chapter 2

American Diabetes Association. (2010). Standards of medical care in diabetes—2010. *Diabetes Care* 33:S11-S61.

Cheskin, L. J., Roberts, C., and Margolis, S. (2010). *Johns Hopkins white papers: Nutrition and weight control for longevity.* New York: MediZine LLC.

Consumer Reports On Health. (2010). Salt: How low should you go? April, 1, 4.

Hensrud, D. (2010). *The Mayo Clinic diet.* Intercourse, PA: Good Books.

The Hershey Company. (n.d.). *Types of chocolate products.* http://www.hersheys.com/nutrition/chocolate.asp (accessed May 24, 2010).

Magee, E. (2009). *Tell me what to eat if I have diabetes.* 3rd ed. Franklin Lakes, NJ: New Page Books.

Mertig, R. G. (2007). *Nurses' guide to teaching diabetes self-management.* New York: Springer Publishing Company, LLC.

U.S. Department of Agriculture. (2005). *The 2005 dietary guidelines for Americans.* http://mypyramid.gov (accessed July 13, 2005).

U.S. Department of Agriculture. (2010). *The 2010 dietary guidelines for Americans.* http://www.cnpp.usda.gov/DGAs 2010-DGACReport.htm (accessed June 21, 2010).

U.S. Food and Drug Administration (n.d.). *How to understand and use nutrition facts labels.* http://www.fda.gov/Food/LabelingNutrition/comsumerinformation/ucm (accessed March 3, 2010).

Warshaw, H. S., and Boderman, K. M. (2001). *Practical carbohydrate counting.* Alexandria, VA: American Diabetes Association.

Chapter 3

Mertig, R. G. (2007). *Nurses' guide to teaching diabetes self-management.* New York: Springer Publishing Company, LLC.

Saudek, C., and Margolis, Si. (2010). *Johns Hopkins white papers: Diabetes.* Baltimore, MD: Johns Hopkins University School of Medicine.

Coltrera, F., and Slon, S. (2010). *Exercise: A program you can live with.* Boston, MA: Harvard University Medical School.

Scheiner, G. (2004). *Think like a pancreas.* New York: Marlowe & Company.

U.S. Department of Agriculture. (2010). *The 2010 dietary guidelines for Americans.* http://www.cnpp.usda.gov/DGAs2010-DGACReport.htm (accessed June 21, 2010).

Skerrett, P. J. (2010). New heart rate estimate for women. *Harvard Heart Letter*, 21 (October): 2, 6.

Chapter 4

American Diabetes Association. (2003). *Insulin therapy in the 21st century.* Alexandria, VA: American Diabetes Association.

Clark, W. L. (2006). Exenatide: From the Gila monster to you. *Diabetes Self-Management* (January–February): 36–40.

DeNoon, D. J. (June 25, 2010). *New type of diabetes drug drops weight and blood sugar.* http://diabetes.webmd.com/news/20100625/new-type-diabetes-drug-drops-weight-blood-sugar?ecd+wnl_dia_070910 (accessed July 9, 2010).

Fox, L. A., Buckloh, L. M., Smith, S. D., Wysocki, T., and Mauras, N. (2005). A randomized controlled trial of insulin pump therapy in young children with type 1 diabetes. *Diabetes Care* 28:1277–81.

Hersch, I. B., Bergenstal, R. M., Parkin, C. G., Wright, E. Jr., and Buse, J. B. (2005). A real-world approach to insulin therapy in primary care practice. *Clinical Diabetes* 23:78–86.

Meece, J. (2006). Dispelling myths and removing barriers about insulin in type 2 diabetes. *Diabetes Educator*, 32(January–February, Suppl. no. 1): 95–175.

Mertig, R. G. (2007). *Nurses' guide to teaching diabetes self-management*. New York: Springer Publishing Company, LLC.

Peyrot, M. (2005). Resistance to insulin therapy among patients and providers. *Diabetes Care* 28(November 7): 2673-79.

Chapter 5

American Diabetes Association. (n.d.). How to administer glucogon [Video]. www.diabetes.org/type-1-diabetes/hypogly-cemia.jsp (accessed October 2, 2010).

American Diabetes Association. (2003). *Insulin therapy in the 21st century*. Alexandria, VA: American Diabetes Association.

American Diabetes Association. (2010). Standards of medical care in diabetes—2010. *Diabetes Care* 33:S11-S61.

Garg, S., Schwartz, S., and Edelman, S. (2004). Improved glucose excursions using an implantable real-time continuous glucose sensor in adults with type 1 diabetes. *Diabetes Care* 27:734-8.

Mendosa, D. (2010). *Blood glucose meters*. http://www.mendosa.com/meters.htm (accessed July 2, 2010).

Mertig, R. G. (2007). *Nurses' guide to teaching diabetes self-management*. New York: Springer Publishing Company, LLC.

Ruhl, J. (2008). *What they don't tell you about diabetes*. Turner Falls, MA: Technion Books.

Scheiner, G. (2004). *Think like a pancreas*. New York: Marlowe & Company.

Chapter 6

Centers for Disease Control and Prevention. (2008). *National diabetes fact sheet, 2007*. http://www.cdc.gov/diabetes (accessed February 15, 2010).

Collazo-Clavell, M. (2009). *Mayo Clinic: The essential diabetes book*. New York: Time, Inc.

Saudek, C., and Margolis, S. (2010). *Johns Hopkins white papers: Diabetes*. Baltimore, MD: Johns Hopkins University School of Medicine.

Chapter 7

American Diabetes Association. (n.d.). *What is gestational diabetes?* http://www.diabetes.org/diabetes-basic/gestational/what-is-gestational-diabetes.html (accessed July 20, 2010).

American Diabetes Association. (2010). Standards of medical care in diabetes—2010. *Diabetes Care* 33:S11-S61.

Barbour, L. A., & Friedman, J. E. (March 6, 2003). *Management of diabetes in pregnancy.*http://mdtext.com/diabetes/diabetes36/diabetes36.htm (accessed March 11, 2006).

Clausen, T. D., Mathiesen, E., Ekbom, P., Hellmuth, E., Mandrup-Poulsen, T., and Damm, P. (2005). Poor pregnancy outcome in women with type 2 diabetes. *Diabetes Care* 28:323-8.

Dabelea, D., Snell-Bergeon, J. K., Hartsfield, C. L., Bischoff, K. J., Hamman, R. F., and McDuffie, R. S. (2005). Increasing prevalence of gestational diabetes mellitus (GDM) over time and by birth cohort. *Diabetes Care* 28:579-84.

Jovanovic, L. (2009). *Medical management of pregnancy complicated by diabetes.* Alexandria, VA: American Diabetes Association.

Mertig, R. G. (2007). *Nurses' guide to teaching diabetes self-management.* New York: Springer Publishing Company, LLC.

Chapter 8

American Diabetes Association. (n.d.-a). *Anger.* http://www.diabetes.org/living-with-diabetes/complications/mental-health/anger.html (accessed September 20, 1010).

American Diabetes Association. (n.d.-b). *Depression.* http://www.diabetes.org/living-with-diabetes/complications/mental-health/depression.html (accessed September 21, 2010).

American Diabetes Association. (n.d.-c). *Stress.* http://www.diabetes.org/living-with-diabetes/complications/stress.html (accessed September 17, 2010).

U.S. National Library of Medicine and National Institutes of Health. (n.d.) *Depression.* http://www.nlm.nih.gov/medlineplus/depression.html (accessed September 23, 2010).

Chapter 9

American Association of Diabetes Educators. (n.d.). *Definitions, diabetes education, diabetes educator.* http://www.diabetes educator.org/DiabetesEducation/Definitions.html (accessed September 2, 2010).

American Diabetes Association. (2010). Standards of medical care in diabetes–2010. *Diabetes Care* 33:S11-S61.

Lorig, K. R., and Halsted, R. H. (2003). Self-management education: History, definition, outcomes, mechanisms. *Annals of Behavioral Medicine* 26(1): 1-7.

Mertig, R. G. (2007). *Nurses' guide to teaching diabetes self-management.* New York: Springer Publishing Company, LLC.

Chapter 10

Rubin, R. R. (n.d.). *Tips for really helping a person who has diabetes.* http://www.diabetes.org/livingwithdiabetes/connect-with-others/support (accessed September 16, 2010).

Polonski, W. (n.d.). *Diabetes etiquette for people who don't have diabetes.* http://behavioraldiabetesinstitute.org/downloads/Etiquette-Card.pdf (accessed September 4, 2010).

Chapter 11

American Diabetes Association. (2010). Standards of medical care in diabetes–2010. *Diabetes Care* 33:S11-S61.

Feste, C. (1995). *The physician within: A step-by-step guide to the motivation you need to meet any health challenge.* New York: Henry Holt.

Feste, C. (2004). *365 Daily meditations for people with diabetes.* Alexandria, VA: American Diabetes Association.

Feste, C. (2007). *Tips and tales from 50 years with diabetes.* Eustis, FL: SPS Publications.

Index